There are so many benefits to becoming a triathlete—maintaining a healthy lifestyl[e], confidence in yourself, accomplishing personal goals and meeting some incredible people along the way. The sport of triathlon is a journey and this book is a great resource to guide you.

—*Mark Wilson, Race Director of HITS Triathlon Series*

This book is a must-read textbook for the success of all new triathletes. For established athletes, the priceless "pro" tips and information are critical for ramping up their efficiency and effectiveness to reach a new personal best.

—*Frank Sole, Masters Swim Coach, Sole Swim Solutions*

7 WEEKS TO A TRIATHLON

BRETT STEWART AND LEWIS ELLIOT

THE COMPLETE DAY-BY-DAY PROGRAM TO TRAIN FOR YOUR FIRST RACE OR IMPROVE YOUR FASTEST TIME

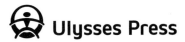
Ulysses Press

Published in the United States by
ULYSSES PRESS
P.O. Box 3440
Berkeley, CA 94703
www.ulyssespress.com

ISBN13: 978-1-61243-096-6
Library of Congress Control Number 2012940417

Printed in the United States by Bang Printing

10 9 8 7 6 5 4 3 2 1

Acquisitions Editor: Keith Riegert
Managing Editor: Claire Chun
Editors: Lauren Harrison, Lily Chou
Index: Sayre Van Young
Cover design: what!design @ whatweb.com
Interior photographs: © Rapt Productions except on page 4 © jbor/shutterstock.com; page 12
    © Joseph Courtney; page 37 © Brett Stewart; page 42 © stemack/shutterstock.com; page 44
    © Jim Larson/shutterstock.com; page 52 © Joseph Courtney; page 88 © jbor/shutterstock.com; page 131
    © Joseph Courtney; page 142 (top) © Kristen Stewart, (bottom) © Joseph Courtney
Front cover photographs: runner © Maridav/shutterstock.com, biker © Stefan Schurr/shutterstock.com,
    Swimmer © AISPIX/shutterstock.com
Back cover photograph: © jbor/shutterstock.com
Models: Austin Akre, Mary J. Gines, Brett Stewart

Distributed by Publishers Group West

Please Note

This book has been written and published strictly for informational purposes, and in no way should be used as a substitute for consultation with health care professionals. You should not consider educational material herein to be the practice of medicine or to replace consultation with a physician or other medical practitioner. The authors and publisher are providing you with information in this work so that you can have the knowledge and can choose, at your own risk, to act on that knowledge. The authors and publisher also urge all readers to be aware of their health status and to consult health care professionals before beginning any health program.

This book is independently authored and published and no sponsorship or endorsement of this book by, and no affiliation with, any trademarked events, brands or other products mentioned or pictured within is claimed or suggested. All trademarks that appear in this book belong to their respective owners and are used here for informational purposes only. The authors and publisher encourage readers to patronize the quality events, brands and other products mentioned and pictured in this book.

In memory of Stephanie Elliot
1953–2003
For your support, encouragement and love, even when a desirable outcome seemed far from likely. We're working tirelessly at living life every day and to find a cure in your memory.

Table of Contents

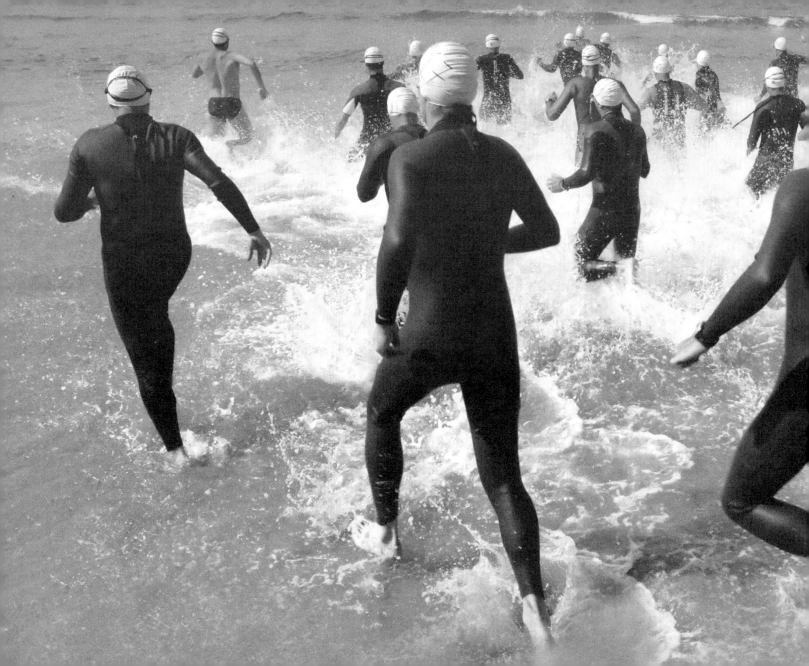

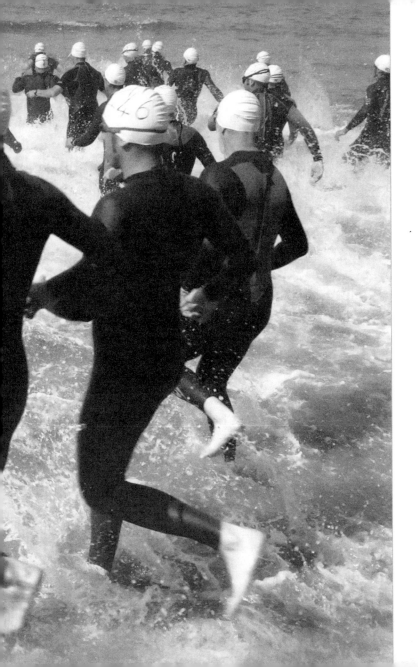

PART 1: OVERVIEW

Introduction

The sunlight begins to glint through the tallest of the pines rimming a pristine New England lake, illuminating the thick layer of haze that's slowly releasing its grip on the water and providing glimpses through to the sapphire below. Standing on the edge of a quiet dock, the moist wood slippery under bare feet, the solitary athlete absorbs a view that's all at once majestic and ephemeral as the day arrives.

As you dip your toe, the summery warmth of the water dispels any allusion to fall as more colors continue to appear in the water; neon orange and lime green orbs now bob within feet of each other and within minutes the area directly in front of the dock has been transformed into a floating Mardi Gras parade awash with bright and garish colors.

It's now your turn to take the plunge, adding the color of your swim cap to the dots floating just above the surface. You hit the water and feel the lake grip at your wetsuit, and the sparkling water washes over your face as you bob gently, buoyant from the neoprene and your legs treading water below you. All those thoughts of the race yet to unfold that ran through your head while standing on the dock fade from your mind as you focus on the task at hand. Weeks of training and planning have prepared for this one moment. The millions of thoughts ranging from conditions to nutrition, gear to competition all dissipate like the haze over the water. You are confident in your preparation. You are confident in your ability and you are ready to race right here, right now. The only thought that sticks in your mind is to keep moving forward: in the water, on the bike and during the run.

All at once the enormity of the day reveals itself in your mind: swimming side by side with hundreds of other athletes all vying for position, a washing machine of flailing arms and legs stretched out over a thousand meters in open water, before returning to shore and rapidly switching gears—literally—by shedding your swimming gear and transforming into a cyclist for the next stage of the day's competition. Through the twists and turns, speedy downhills and grueling ascents, the steely determination to pass or be passed overtakes the next two hours of exhausting effort as you push your quads to their limit and keep turning the cranks with every ounce of energy you have left. Returning to transition is a blur of rapid motion, a cacophony of sounds as the announcer whips the crowd into a frenzy; friends and family scream your name as you perform a coordinated dance of returning your bike back to its perch on the rack while ripping off your helmet and bike shoes and applying the required gear for the run. The final challenge between you and the finish line, the run is where mental and physical strength are paramount—pushing your body through barriers of exhaustion toward the euphoric highs as you power around the course, one foot in front of the other, until…

You finish the day as a newer version of yourself—you will have been transformed into a *triathlete*.

> Many people settle for things in life. They settle for a crappy job, marriage, friends, food, place to live and overall fitness and health. Those who desire more, or those who want more out of life than a drive-thru window and boring sitcom, will choose triathlon or an activity that makes them happy—an activity that will change their life.
> —Nick Clark, Clark Endurance

How Did I Get Here?

Hi, I'm Brett. Running was never my thing. I wasn't fast and surely didn't have much in the way of endurance, but at least I was a lousy swimmer too. It's easy to see how I'd become a triathlete with a background like that, right? Prior to my first triathlon, the last time I'd ridden a road bike was when I was 15 years old—nearly 20 years earlier.

At the age of 34, most life-altering changes are spawned by one stark, defining moment. A guy might lose his job and decide to hike the Appalachian Trail. A woman may get divorced, devote herself to yoga and open her own studio. In my case, it was an anecdotal comment by my friend Chris Goggin, who told me how impressed he was that a mutual friend, Matt Perkins, had recently completed his first triathlon. I was immediately awestruck. Prior to Matt tackling that Winding Trails event, I knew exactly zero people who had ever competed in a triathlon. Suddenly, a new door opened and completing a triathlon seemed *somewhat* possible. I say "somewhat" because the longest I'd ever run was 2 miles, with the aforementioned Chris Goggin, in my first race ever—a little duathlon on the Connecticut shoreline in 2004.

After running close to a half mile and walking the rest, the bike portion of that first race was spent chasing after a dropped water bottle, fixing my chain that was continually falling off and pushing my sad excuse for a mountain bike up anything that resembled a hill. The final insult was another run of 2 miles once I'd parked the bike, and I was dreading every step until something strange happened: I heard the crowd, saw my family and observed the other competitors doing something nearly unbelievable to my fatigued mind—they were enjoying themselves! I let the energy and emotion wash over me for a moment, then figured, "What the hell? I'm here, I'm already tired and sweaty—why not try to have some fun?" And I did.

In my very first multisport event I learned the lessons of the highs and lows of endurance racing, and that knowledge has served me well for the better part of a decade. The birth of my children and wedding day (the second one) aside, crossing that finish line was one of the best moments of my life. Immediately afterward over coffee and a bagel, Chris and I planned our next event— we were going to do a triathlon ourselves.

The story on pages 7 and 8 was based on the memory of my first triathlon in 2005, the Timberman Short Course at Lake Winnipesaukee in New Hampshire. The reason I introduced myself is to set my multisport

> This sport called triathlon becomes a part of you. You start to plan your entire year around sprint, international, half iron- or full iron-distance races. Your vacations become racing, and you start to realize that this could become a life-long adventure.
> —Nick Clark, Clark Endurance

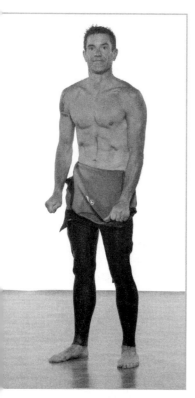

expertise apart from that of my coauthor, Lewis Elliot, a professional triathlete. While I'm an experienced triathlete and extremely passionate about the sport, my forte is getting first-timers into it through education and training to promote comfort and confidence. As a trainer, coach and tri-race director, I've had the opportunity to introduce hundreds of "newbies" to the sport of triathlon and have been blessed to train clients for events ranging from finishing their first sprint tri all the way up to setting a new ultra-distance personal best.

When cofounding the ESPN Triathlon Team back in 2005 with Michael DeAngelo and Nicole Greene, it was immediately apparent to us that so many athletes knew so little about the sport of triathlon, whether it be a lack of knowledge about equipment, training, race format or even signing up for their first race. Triathlon is not a sport where you just show up and start racing—it all starts with learning the basics. This book is dedicated to educating new athletes getting into the sport (yeah, you're called a "newbie"), and also to train experienced triathletes to get to the next level with pro tips plucked from Lewis's bag of tricks. So, whether you're interested in "tri-ing" for yourself or are already hooked on multisport, this book has something for athletes of all levels.

About the Book

Even if you're not an accomplished swimmer, biker or runner, becoming a triathlete is a life-changing accomplishment that everyone can attain. The multisport community is filled with competitors of every age, height, weight and athletic ability. I've had the honor of competing alongside blind triathletes, athletes missing limbs and heroes who were injured in battle, I've been passed on the bike by women double my age and twice my size, and even been humbled by an octogenarian who passed me within sight of the finish line during a long-distance race. Triathlon is truly a sport for everyone.

Throughout the pages of this book we've assembled tips, tricks and techniques to help you survive your first triathlon or gain more insight into becoming even faster on the course.

Part I introduces the sport of triathlon: the history, individual race distances and frequently asked questions. "Getting Started in Triathlon" on page 26 covers everything a first-timer needs to know before they take the plunge at their first race. "Taking It to the Next Level" on page 41 delivers a wealth of information in the form of 35 pro-quality tips to help experienced triathletes improve their technique and times.

Part II contains two training programs. The first is the seven-week Beginner program, which covers all the basics, from getting in the water for the first time to running a solid 5k to completing your first sprint or Olympic-distance triathlon. Complete with tips, tricks and advice to make the sport less daunting, this program has been developed for the first-timer or novice who wants to learn more to be able to truly enjoy the sport of triathlon.

The Advanced program is designed for the experienced multisport athlete to take their fitness and racing to the next level. Whether your goal is racing a long course or ultra distance, this section contains the same training used by top triathletes to help transform your body and meet your goals.

Part III explains the importance of cross-training for triathlon success and describes over two dozen different exercises, stretches and drills to strengthen your body, build endurance and flexibility, and improve your triathlon results.

Here you'll also find stretches and warm-ups for training, cross-training and on race day. Finally, we've compiled a glossary of triathlon terms to help beginners figure out what all this triathlon lingo really means!

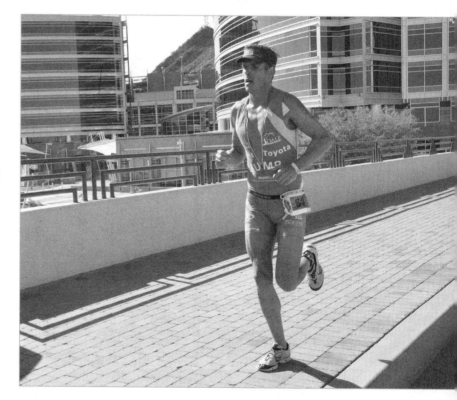

Additional material that didn't make it into the book, as well as an online forum packed with additional tips and advice from athletes just like you, can be found on www.7weekstofitness.com. Log on and share your stories about becoming a triathlete!

How to Use This Book

Whether this is your first or fiftieth triathlon, there are nuggets of information everywhere in the book, from the "Triathlon Terms" on page 129 to the FAQs, programs, tips…well, you get the idea. Experienced triathletes will find a wealth of helpful techniques in the pro tips starting on page 41, and will most likely learn quite a bit in even the beginner sections. This book is designed for the experienced triathlete to hand to their spouse and friends so they can understand and appreciate the sport better, as well as for athletes who are excited to try triathlon for the first time. You don't have to absorb it all at once. Just like the sport of triathlon itself, it takes some time and patience to learn all you can.

We've developed training programs that are significantly different from those you'll find in some other publications or online, specifically the way the programs are written. We don't throw a list of 5x100, 80% VO_2 max for you to try to translate, but we explain what every workout should entail as if you were talking to a coach. While we can't be right next to everyone at the pool or out on the bike, we put in as much effort as possible to speak to you as if we were. You can bet we would be if we could.

Enjoy the book, and we hope you fall in love with this crazy sport of triathlon.

> The individual sports of swimming, biking and running are fantastic in their own right, but there's something about putting them all together that changes the way we feel about ourselves and the way we feel about the sport of triathlon.
> —Mark H. Wilson, Race Director of HITS Triathlon Series

What Is a Triathlon?

By its most basic definition, a triathlon is an event involving the completion of three back-to-back endurance events, typically swimming, cycling and running over various distances.

According to most triathletes (or their significant others), "Triathlon is some form of mind-altering hallucinogenic drug that starts innocently enough—dabble with a sprint distance here, a few brick workouts there—until it becomes an all-encompassing addiction that makes normally sound-minded individuals swap their baggy sweatpants for body-clinging suits and eventually spirals out of control, culminating in men with shaved legs and women who will gladly run over slower shoppers with a cart to get to the checkout line first."

> **Fact: You will not become efficient at swimming, biking or running overnight. This is NOT an easy sport.**
> —Nick Clark, Clark Endurance

While there may be some truth in the above definition, there's a much softer side to becoming a triathlete—the camaraderie, support and friendship that are developed while training and racing with others are a large part of the allure. Meeting and training with like-minded athletes makes triathlon less of an individual sport and much more of a community. Because of this, triathlon teams and clubs can be found in nearly every spot around the globe.

Our definition of triathlon is simple: *competition*. Before you make the decision to train for your first triathlon, you're competing against your fears. If you don't overcome them, you've already lost.

Once you've made the commitment to start training, you're competing against your ability: The swim is too hard, the bike course is too long and you're exhausted during the run. Again, these are obstacles to becoming a multisport athlete, and one by one you must overcome each of them.

The first time you dip your toes in the water at an event, you're competing with a rush of adrenaline, fear of the unknown and 1.2 million thoughts about what that race may bring. You may also be competing with a sticky zipper on a wetsuit, a wobbly wheel on the bike or laces that just won't stay tied on the run.

As you become more experienced, the competition shifts to the guy or gal next to you, with the realization that they may very well stand between you and the podium. It's you versus them, and the rivalry, while good-natured, is intense from the moment the gun sounds until the finish line.

The sport of triathlon is always a competition: against the elements, your physical ability, your race readiness, your choice of gear. Most importantly, it's always a race against time.

The History of Triathlon

Triathlon is one of the most widely known multisport races, timed athletic competitions consisting of a series of different disciplines that are performed back to back. There are others of relative prominence: duathlon (run, bike, run), aquathlon (swim, run) and aquabike

IRONMAN AND IRONMAN©

Tell any non-triathlete you're training for a triathlon and the first three questions they ask will invariably be: *"You're doing a 'real' one?" "Isn't that in Hawaii?" "Don't you bike a hundred miles and then run a marathon after you swam like 5 miles?"*

Most people understand it's a race composed of swimming, biking and running (although they usually get the order wrong), but the most common misconception is that every triathlon takes place in Hawaii and is the "real" distance. Simply put, non-athletes mistake every triathlon with the Ironman World Championships in Kona. This is akin to calling every car a '67 Corvette 427 or saying every running race is the Boston Marathon.

What many non-triathletes also probably don't understand is that "Ironman" and "Ironman Triathlon" are trademarks of World Triathlon Corporation (WTC), by far the most recognized brand in triathlon events, and are a specific brand of triathlon held all over the world. While it's common to refer to a 140.6-mile triathlon as Ironman-distance or an "Ironman," the name is only official if it's an event put on by the WTC. All other 140.6-mile triathlons are "Iron distance," or the more correct term, "ultra distance."

spotty history of the sport throughout the '20s, and a 1934 article touts "Les Trois Sports" featuring a 200-meter swim, a 10-kilometer bike competition and a 1200-meter run, although it's not entirely clear if they were performed back to back in rapid succession as multisport events are today.

Currently, there are several larger organizations that host multiple events each year:

- XTERRA, which puts on off-road triathlons worldwide

- HITS Triathlon Series

- 5150 (owned by WTC), which has events in both the U.S. and internationally

- Revolution 3

- Amica 19.7

- Tri Rock

While this new breed of multisport seemed to sputter into relative obscurity in Europe, the modern version of the sport now known as triathlon was born in San Diego, California. On September 24, 1974, the San Diego Track and Field Club staged a fledgling event at Mission Bay consisting of a 5.3-mile run, a 5-mile cycle race and a 600-yard swim in Mission Bay. The race was originally created as an alternative to the rigors of track-based training and was only planned to contain two events—a

(swim, bike), to name a few. Early versions of multisport competitions were even more diverse.

Multisport events were held as early as 1902 in France, composed of running, cycling and canoeing. In 1920, the first documented race consisting of running, cycling and swimming took place in northeastern France along the river Marne. Newspaper articles chronicle the

Event	Swim	Bike	Run
Open Distance	100 m	3 mi	1 mi
Super (or Ultra) Sprint	400 m	10 km	2.5 km
Sprint	500–750 m	20 km	5 km
Olympic (International, Standard or Short Course)	1.5 km	40 km	10 km
International Long Distance (Double Olympic or O2)	3 km	80 km	20 km
Long Course (70.3, Half Distance)	1.2 mi (1.9 km)	56 mi (90 km)	13.1 mi (21.09 km)
Ultra Distance (140.6, Full Distance)	2.4 mi (3.8 km)	112 mi (180 km)	26.2 mi (42.195 km)

run followed by a swim. Race organizer Jack Johnstone was reluctantly convinced to include the bike portion at the insistence of cyclist Don Shanahan, and the first "modern" triathlon was born: the Mission Bay Triathlon. The word *triathlon* was actually coined by Johnstone, who adapted it from the sport of decathlon.

Well-known and historical triathlons include: Vineman Triathlon (Windsor, California); Silverman Triathlon (Henderson, Nevada); Chicago Triathlon; Malibu Triathlon; Escape from Alcatraz Triathlon; XTERRA Maui World Championships; and St. Anthony's Triathlon (St. Petersburg, Florida).

Triathlon Distances

Any event composed of a swim, bike course and run is a triathlon, and the distances vary considerably, especially for off-road races. Kid's and beginner events are usually super sprint or less, and often feature a pool swim. HITS Triathlon Series created the open distance, geared toward first-timers and beginners; as of this printing, race entry is free. The distances above are recognized by either the governing bodies of the International Triathlon Union (ITU) and USA Triathlon (USAT), or through WTC or HITS Triathlon Series. The ITU accepts a 5% variance in the cycle and run course distances.

Triathlon's Future

"OK, smarty-pants author guys, if triathlon is a sport that anyone can do, why aren't there more family-friendly events?"

Well, it's simple. The challenge associated with triathlon had for many decades been a limiting factor in its growth and somewhat relegated it to a fringe sport for only the fittest athletes, with a disproportionate number of them male. The recent explosion in popularity of the sport has all but erased the barriers to entry for any interested athlete of either gender at any age. The advent of multiple female-only triathlons, development of IronKids for 6- to 15-year-olds and a large number of races featuring two or more distances at an event has helped to make triathlon something for everyone.

Leading the charge in this emerging trend of family-friendly triathlons is a race series that features five different race distances over a weekend called HITS Triathlon Series, whose tagline is literally "A Distance for Everyone." The open division at this race series doesn't just lower the barrier to entry, it blows the doors wide open by making it free for novices and first-timers to compete. You read that right: free. Even shorter than a super sprint in distance, the open category is ideal for those who never thought they'd be able to participate in a triathlon.

The structure of holding five different race lengths over one weekend allows families with one or more athletes to watch and support each other before their events begin. Mom and Dad can watch their child race the open, Mom can race the Olympic later that day and Dad can race the long course or ultra on Sunday! Forward-thinking race organizations like HITS Triathlon Series show that the individual disciplines of triathlon— swim, bike and run—have changed very little from the sport's humble beginnings, and innovative event organizers can build on the foundation of triathlon and the passion of millions of fans around the globe by creating events that are more family-, fan- and participant-friendly. The future of triathlon is about to be rewritten as truly a distance for everyone!

> **Swimming, biking, running, pace, power output, cadence, stroke, gear, chafing... all these things that you think about during an event must mean you're crazy or obsessed. You're a triathlete—and that means you're both!**

Why Triathlon?

Why do people climb mountains? The common answer is "because they were there," and of course the real answer lies deeper than that. The primal desire to challenge your mind and body propels athletes to dig deep and overcome any obstacle placed in front of them. The allure of multisport draws athletes in with a simple question: "I wonder if I could do that?" With over 2.4 million triathlon participants in 2011, approximately 35 percent of them first-timers, it's a question asked—and answered—by millions each year.

Triathlon—and more specifically, triathlon training—is a challenge for any athlete that improves their physical conditioning, strength, flexibility, agility, visual acuity and endurance for any other sport. Becoming a triathlete can be considered the ultimate cross-training; splitting the workouts between swimming, cycling and running balances out the strain on any particular muscle group while consistently taxing your body in a multitude of ways. Triathlon is all about taking your fitness to the next level, and is the ultimate in functional athletic training. "Bricks" (see "Triathlon Terms" on page 129) are an all-in-one cross-training workout through two of the disciplines and can be regarded as the ultimate cardio and adrenaline rush wrapped up into a single exercise regimen.

Triathlon training is responsible for more lean, strong and fast physiques than every fitness DVD in the world combined (OK, we made this up, but hopefully you get the point). If you're picking a sport to lose weight and get stronger and significantly fitter, triathlon is it!

Aside from the health benefits, the sport of triathlon fosters a unique community of athletes who train together, share tips, tricks and techniques, and support each other before and after races—and try their damnedest to beat each other on the race course. The explosion of triathlon teams speaks to the camaraderie that's developed between athletes of all abilities and adrenaline junkies who love to train together, hang out afterward and share stories or training plans. Search online for teams or groups in your area, inquire at a local bike shop or check out Facebook. You'll be happy you did.

Let's not forget the aspect of pure, unbridled adrenaline that an athlete feels when competing in a race, whether it's a 5k or an ultra distance triathlon. The dopamine-producing endorphins are only compounded by competition among other athletes as you race from discipline to discipline, transitioning from swimming to biking to running to the peak of your ability. Don't let anyone tell you any differently: The sport of triathlon is like a drug to many, but with very positive side effects!

> Every time you show up at a triathlon, you only have one chance to race this course; the changing weather conditions, your fitness level, your preparedness and mental state are all variables. Even if it's a course you have raced hundreds of times—every race is a completely new experience.

Frequently Asked Questions

Whether you're getting ready to tackle your first triathlon or want to pick up some tips from the pros, these FAQs cover some of the most common questions asked by newbies and some great pointers for the experienced triathlete.

Q. What's the best tip you can give to someone interested in getting into triathlon?

A. Volunteer at an event. Spectating is a good way to get the feel for what a triathlon looks like outside the ropes, but when you volunteer you're part of the action and have your finger directly on the pulse of the event. You can pick up a ton of useful tips by watching and listening to the athletes around you. Arrive early and spend a good deal of time in the transition area, the heart of any triathlon. If the event you're volunteering at gives discounts or free entry to a future race, you're off to a flying start!

Q. I'm a first-timer. Can I really do a triathlon?

A. Yes. All potential athletes should have a complete physical examination prior to beginning training for a triathlon. Provided that your physician has approved your participation, most amateurs will be able to complete a sprint distance triathlon (0.75k or 0.5-mile swim; 20k or 12-mile bike; 5k or 3.1-mile run) in 1.5 to 3 hours. Fit, healthy individuals should be able to prepare adequately to complete these distances with a minimum of seven weeks training. If that distance seems daunting, look for a shorter "open" or super-sprint distance for your first race.

Q. I'm new to triathlon. Do I need a coach?

A. Almost all athletes can benefit from a coach. Newer triathletes should join a triathlon group or club and start learning from other athletes; training with faster and more experienced triathletes is the quickest way to get better. If at some point along the way a triathlon coach fits into your budget, then it's definitely not a bad idea. Aspiring triathletes without a swimming background should definitely get a swim coach and join a master's swim team. Swimming is one area where all the work in the world won't make you better without a good coach helping you with your technique. Remember that every triathlon coach will have different philosophies toward how to prepare for your races, and each has their own methods to make you faster. It's important that you can talk with your coach about your ideas, feelings and experiences so they have vital information that can help guide you through the tough decisions while pursuing triathlon success.

Q. I've never done a triathlon, but one day I want to do a long course or ultra distance triathlon. Should I just sign up for a race of that distance a year down the road and start a training plan?

A. While it's definitely possible to train for a long-distance event as your first triathlon, it's not recommended, as there are many nuances to racing a triathlon that need to be experienced in an actual race. If your goal is to go from newbie triathlete to doing a long course or ultra distance triathlon in one year, which is an extremely aggressive time frame, then it's recommended that you sign up for shorter triathlons before your long-distance event. At every race you compete in, whether it be a 5k running race or an open-water swim, you'll learn something new. A solid plan is to compete in one race a month for the next 12 months in preparation for a long-distance triathlon, getting progressively longer in distance as you get closer to your target race. See "Progressing in Races" on page 40.

Q. I go to the local races and all the other triathletes have aero bike frames, disc and deep-dish wheels, and aero helmets. Do I need this equipment to compete?

A. For a new triathlete, going to events can be a little intimidating and overwhelming for a variety of reasons. The equipment most triathletes purchase early on often borders on ridiculous. You don't need any of the expensive aerodynamic gear to successfully compete and progress in the sport. It's fun if you have the extra money to get a little bit of "free speed." See page 47 for how to get the most bang for your buck when it comes to buying some speed.

Q. I've been training hard for a while now and my results seem to have hit a plateau. I don't feel tired or overtrained, so how do I break through and get to a new level?

A. Most of the time when an athlete reaches a plateau, it's a good idea to take a step back and recover, and then build back up again. The other likely possibility is that an athlete is approaching their reasonable potential with the current stimulus and needs to start changing things up a bit. A good plan would be to identify your weaknesses as a triathlete. For example, you may have no swimming background and therefore have slower swim splits, or you may be very skinny and could benefit from full-body cross-training. Whatever you discover, identify that weakness, and for the next seven weeks focus on that area more than you have before. Continue your regular swim/bike/run training while putting more effort on strengthening that weakness and you'll start to see positive gains, eventually breaking through that plateau.

Q. I want to do an Ironman triathlon, but I want the easiest course and to get a really fast time. Which one should I do?

A. Historically, the races in Europe are the fastest. Ironman Germany, Iron-distance Roth Challenge, Ironman Austria—these are the races where the top pros are breaking the eight-hour barrier. This translates to faster times for your everyday triathlete. Assuming you don't want to travel to Europe, Ironman Arizona can be a very fast course, as can Ironman Florida. Both being in the fall, their conditions are usually mild and they're both relatively flat. Of course, conditions can have a big effect on finishing times; if it's raining and cold or windy, the times will be slower across the board.

Q. Will those elastic or speed-lace things make me any faster in a triathlon?

A. Many top triathletes view the triathlon as five events: swim, T1, bike, T2, run. Because triathlon measures total time, it's imperative that a competitive triathlete moves through transition as quickly as possible. Elastic or "speed laces" are designed to speed up that process and save you valuable seconds, if that's what you're after. There are a few different brands. Find one that works well for you and gives you speedy transitions, and stick with it!

Q. What is the best surface to run on for triathlon training?

A. Generally, athletes should train by running on the same surface they plan to race on, but it can be beneficial to practice and train your body on all surfaces. You may find it nice to do your long run on a trail or dirt path; many have theorized this lower-impact running will have you breaking down less over time, allowing for fewer injuries. Many athletes do minimalist-shoe running on grass or a sports field as part of their training. Track workouts 1 to 2 times a week are a key element of many professionals' training. Tempo or race pace runs can be done on a cinder trail, sidewalk, treadmill or at the track. It's best to be ready for anything you may encounter on race day, so mix up the terrain you run on day to day and week to week.

Q. Time is short with my wife, kids and work. I sleep about 7 hours a night. Should I get up an hour earlier every day to increase my training volume?

A. In most cases this would be a bad idea. For an endurance athlete, sleep is imperative. It's when your body recovers the most from workouts and this is where marked improvements are made. Sleep should almost never be sacrificed long-term for increased training. If you feel you've reached your potential based on the number of hours a week you currently train, you may benefit by restructuring your life slightly to get a little more training in each week. For example, can you commute to work by bike? Perhaps run on your lunch break or buy a bike trainer or treadmill and work out while watching the kids? Another option would be to increase training adaptation by focusing on mainly high-intensity workouts to make the most of the time you have.

> Rest is the key to progressing in training or racing. Any athlete will become apathetic and lethargic if they do not get the appropriate amount of rest. The only way to prevent burnout and overtraining is to listen to your body and back off immediately. Take a couple days off until your muscles start to feel fresh again.
> —Mark H. Wilson, Race Director of HITS Triathlon Series

Q. I live in a cold climate. What is the best form of cross-training for triathlon during the off-season?

A. Despite triathlon being a combination of three different sports, it's still a fairly linear activity and does not necessarily involve supporting muscles for twisting and changing direction like most ball sports do. In order to maintain a high level of fitness and keep from burning out by doing the same training and athletics 12 months a year, participate in sports like basketball, tennis, indoor or outdoor soccer, bodyweight exercises (like those found in the cross-training workouts on page 92), weight lifting and racquetball. Each of these work kinesthetic awareness as well as balance, and build strength, flexibility and agility for a more universal and less linear muscular structure. It's important, however, to be very careful when starting different sports after a triathlon season as it takes a while for your body to adapt. Taking some time off from triathlon training will keep you from getting stale in your workouts and help you enjoy other sports while staying in top shape between seasons.

Q. Recently I've been under the weather. Should I keep training or rest until I feel better?

A. The old rule of thumb is to work out if symptoms are above the neck, rest if they're below the neck. Usually athletes can train through a basic head cold, but it's a good idea to take it easy. Maybe go 75% in intensity and duration of your normal scheduled workout. Usually when we get sick, our body is sending us messages: more rest, better nutrition and reduced stress. It's important that all athletes make an effort to listen!

Getting Started in Triathlon

A triathlon is a work in progress from the moment you wake up on race day until you cross the finish line—nothing is ever guaranteed.

So, You're Going to Participate in Your First Triathlon?

Triathlons are exciting, fun and challenging for athletes of all levels. From the shortest kid's race to ultra distance events, there's a race that's right for everyone. Remember, every single multisport athlete was a newbie at some point, and nearly every single experienced triathlete will fondly remember their first time and how exciting, frustrating, exhilarating and maddeningly complicated it seemed—and how much they loved every second of it. Don't be afraid to ask questions of experienced triathletes; you can even ask advice of people around you in transition pre-race.

Any triathlon can be broken down into three pieces: the athlete, the gear and the course/event.

The Athlete

Remember, a strong body starts with a strong mind. If you're holding this book in your hands (guess what—you are!), there's an extremely good chance that you can complete a triathlon; nearly anyone can.

Look at a triathlon like this:

- Any combination of freestyle, breast stroke, dog paddle and backstroke can be used to complete the swim.

- During the bike leg, you can go as slow as you need to and even walk your bike up hills if necessary.

- The run? That can be a walk/jog/run/waddle to the finish line.

See? Triathlons don't sound so hard, especially when you get the foolish thought out of your head that you can't do it.

WHAT'S YOUR RACE GOAL?

During the race you'll have plenty of time alone with your thoughts; heck, your mind will wander all over the place. If you've set a goal, you'll have something to keep you focused. For your first triathlon, it's a mistake to make any time-specific goals. It's also a mistake to look at other people at the starting line and say, "I bet I can finish before her/him." Your first triathlon is a competition with you against the course, all while on the clock.

For your first triathlon, you really need to savor the experience, and your only goal should be to finish the race and fall in love with the sport. Hopefully, there will be a lot of other races in your future for you to go faster or finish higher up on the leaderboard!

ENDORPHIN ROLLER COASTER: THE HIGHS AND LOWS

Much has been said about "hitting the wall" in a marathon at or around the 20-mile mark, and there may be some truth to it as a physical limitation for some, but for the most part it's entirely mental. In any endurance event, your mind will be your best friend and your worst enemy—all in the span of a few minutes. There'll be amazing highs where your heart will flow with boundless love for the spectators or an aid station worker handing you a cup of water, followed immediately by feelings of self loathing and outright anger toward other competitors, the course or that floppy shoe lace that's driving you insane. The worst part? You'll have no idea when it'll happen. Even during the best race of your life, as you push your body, your mind will fluctuate between light and dark. These highs and lows are relatively universal in endurance racing, so you're not going nuts if you alternate between Dr. Jekyll and Mr. Hyde out on the course.

The best way to deal with these waves is to enjoy the highs and be careful not to push yourself too hard while you're feeling like a superhero. When the lows come, you need to breathe deeply, relax and remind your neurons who's in charge. If the thought of quitting pops into your head, just remember how far you've come and how bummed you'll be later if you bow out now.

DON'T FEAR THE SWIM

For a lot of people, the swim can be the most frightening leg. Simply put, during the swim, stopping to rest is not always an option. All triathlons have lifeguards and aid personnel in kayaks or boats during the swim leg to help you if you're truly in need. You can hang on kayaks, boats, docks or sides of the pool to catch your breath if necessary, as long as you do not propel yourself forward. During the swim, you can use any stroke that you feel comfortable with; while freestyle is the most efficient to cut through the water, alternating between breast and backstroke will allow you to breathe more easily.

Above all, stay as calm as you possibly can in the water for optimal swim success.

The amount of time you spend in the water is about one-fifth of the race, so you don't want to waste all your energy by thrashing in the water because of nerves. In order to swim efficiently, you need to be relaxed and develop an even rhythm with your strokes and kicks. If you fight the water, it'll only slow you down; your goal is to cut through the water as efficiently as possible.

When you first jump into the water, it may be a bit of a shock. Slowly tread water and breathe deeply while you get used to the water temperature and relax. It's very important to be comfortable in the water and not panic if you get kicked, have a cramp or get tired. If you panic in the water, you make it much more difficult for yourself to get control of the situation.

> *TIP:* Need some confidence in the water? A wetsuit will make you more buoyant and streamlined. It's important that you practice with a wetsuit because the constricting feeling may exacerbate feelings of having difficulty breathing; this is perfectly normal and goes away as you calm down and get comfortable.

Before you get into the water, make sure you spot exactly where you'll be exiting the water and what direction to run to get to transition. There will be signs and volunteers to point you in the right direction, and it's always more comforting to have your bearings. When you exit the water, you'll be stripping off your cap and goggles, and unzipping the back of your wetsuit—it's easy to get confused about where you're going.

HELL ON WHEELS: THE BIKE COURSE

The most important part of the bike leg in your first triathlon is to be aware of your surroundings and keep yourself under control. There's a big difference between a "bike ride" and a race; there are experienced riders who are blazingly fast and will be tearing by you at high speeds.

The rules of triathlon require you to stay as far right as possible unless you're passing a slower rider. After you've passed, move back to the right when you're clear of that rider. You're never allowed to ride on the left side of the lane if you're not involved in a pass; this means you're "blocking," which is illegal and a danger to yourself and other faster riders behind you. If you're caught blocking by an official, you'll be assessed a time penalty.

Be attentive of other riders; they may not be as courteous as you are, but it's everyone's responsibility to keep themselves and others around them safe. Be aware that even on closed courses there are plenty of hazards,

including potholes, curbs, spectators and even vehicles. Don't ride in fear that something may happen, but make sure you're aware of the possibility and plan how to handle yourself.

THE RUN

Once you've hit transition 2 and head out for the run, the finish line is in sight, literally. Usually the finisher's chute is located near transition, and there's a chance you're running away from it. Whether you're a great runner or not, you still need to pace yourself when you start the run. You should be a little tired (if not totally gassed) by this point, but you can finish as long as you listen to your body. If you need to rest, then walk for a little bit—nearly every triathlete does during one race or another. There's a common point of discussion whether it's actually better or faster to run for 5 to 10 minutes and then walk for 30 seconds to 1 minute. Some people swear that the benefit of resting your legs and lungs far outweighs the time spent walking. Try it out for yourself on training runs and see if it works for you.

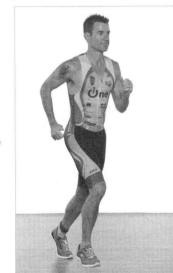

FINISH LINE

If you start to fade during any part of the race, just think about how wonderful it'll feel to cross the finish line. The sense of accomplishment in completing your first triathlon—no matter what your time is—will change your life. You'll officially be a "triathlete," and you'll wear that distinction with pride for the rest of your life. Relish it!

PREPARING PHYSICALLY

Training is very important, and we've created triathlon-specific Beginner (page 56) and Advanced (page 73) programs as well as cross-training exercises, stretches and warm-ups to help you prepare for your first—or fastest—triathlon.

It almost goes without saying that an athlete really needs to be prepared for a triathlon, especially the swim. It's not recommended that anyone sign up for their first triathlon without spending at least a few weeks—minimum—training in a pool. Before the race, you should feel comfortable swimming the same distance as your first race without stopping or putting your feet down. You don't have to swim with perfect form, but for safety's sake you need to be ready for the swim.

The hardest part about swimming longer distances for first-timers is not their form or stroke, it's learning to breathe properly. Don't give up if you're exhausted after trying to swim only one length of the pool; most likely you're not tired, but out of breath from erratic gasping for air. Focus on getting your body high in the water and turning your head to breathe instead of lifting your head each time you need to take a breath. Ask another swimmer for some pointers or talk to a lifeguard at your local pool.

Preparing for a bike race is significantly different from taking your bike out for a ride. It's vital that you pace yourself in all three legs of a triathlon, but that's especially true on the bike as it's the longest section of the day. For efficiency, focus on an even and smooth pedal stroke; you shouldn't feel like you're jabbing at the pedals. Once you're up to a comfortable cruising speed, you can push harder or let off based on how your body feels; just don't push too hard too soon. Having a flat foot at the bottom of the stroke will help you engage your hamstrings on the upstroke to help balance out the effort of your quads on the downstroke.

The run is usually the easiest of the three disciplines to prepare for, bearing in mind that it comes last and you're already going to be fatigued. Like in the biking and swimming legs, your pace is extremely important. A common phrase for beginner triathletes is "Start slow and keep slowing down until you see the finish line—

> *TIP:* During your first race you'll have no barometer as to how hard you can push before failure, so always try to maintain a consistent effort from swim through run. This may be harder than it seems with all the excitement and electricity of the event, but listen to your body and push when you can while staying within your ability.

then run like hell!" The run leg is a great deal easier to moderate your pace, because you can slow down to a walk if you're too fatigued. Remember there's no shame in walking…just try to run if you see a race photographer!

The Gear

All you really need to compete in your first triathlon is a pair of shorts, swim goggles, running shoes and a bike. Your bike is the most critical piece of equipment that you need to be able to count on. Aside from your wetsuit zipper sticking, foggy goggles or your running shoes falling apart, the bike is the only real chance for mechanical problems that could potentially sabotage your race.

YOUR FIRST BIKE

Can you remember getting your first bike as a kid? Shiny, fast and all yours! Well, we hate to spoil your fun, but for your first race you should consider the following.

Road and tri bikes are not cheap; for the most part you really get what you pay for. A mistake that many newbie athletes make is to rush out and buy an "entry-level" bike brand new for $500 to $800, and there's a good chance that they'll outgrow it after a season or two. Build your tri chops up first and save toward buying the right bike at the right time. You'll know it when you get there.

Most triathletes start out with a mountain bike or an older 10- to 12-speed to figure out if they even like

triathlons before buying an expensive road- or tri-bike. If you're planning to use a mountain bike for a road-based triathlon, do yourself a favor and pick up a pair of road tires. If you're using an old road bike, make sure you bring it to a shop to get tuned up and checked out.

If you don't have an older bike of your own laying around the house, you do have several options for your first race:

Borrow one. There's a good chance that one of your friends who talked you into triathlons may have the old bike they started out on or know someone who can loan you one.

Buy a used one at a yard sale or online. This will require some planning and research. You can usually find all the specs and prices online and compare it to what the seller is asking. Finding the proper size is an imperfect science, but since seat posts and handlebars are adjustable, you'll be happy buying close to your ideal size. All major bike companies feature a sizing chart on

BUYING VS. BUILDING

On the surface, building your bike component by component may seem like a good idea; it may even seem cheaper than buying a complete bike. IT ISN'T. Unless you have a lot of time, a full wallet and plenty of hair to tear out when you make a mistake, don't build your own bike. As long as you don't have a race anytime soon and a backup is available, it should be a good learning experience. There are plenty of resources online to confuse, er, help you put it back together.

their websites for each model, so compare the bike for sale to your body dimensions according to their chart. The most important number to check is the "stand-over" height, the distance from the top bar to the ground; this should closely match your inseam (pant leg) size. Unless you're very small, stay away from a 650cm-wheel bike and go with the traditional 700cm wheel. Ask an experienced triathlete for advice before you buy; a good place to start would be an online forum or a local tri club. Try to find a bike in good condition that's 3 to 5 years old—it'll be cheap enough to afford and most likely the components will still be in good-enough shape to use for a while. Talk the seller down by at least $75 if the bike needs a tune-up, then bring it to a shop to get it safety checked and lubed.

CHANGING A FLAT TIRE

If you've never changed a tube before, Murphy's Law is just waiting for the most inopportune time to strike. Changing a flat during a race for the first time is a recipe for disaster, and not only will you lose a great deal of time trying to figure it out on the fly, you possibly won't finish the race. With race entry being rather expensive, not learning to change a four dollar tube can result in wasting over a hundred dollars in entry fees and not even get to the end of the race. Remember, if you do not complete any single leg in a triathlon you're not permitted to continue, and your day is over. At www.7weekstofitness.com we have some helpful links to videos and guidelines to make changing a flat and other simple bike maintenance less of a mystery.

Rent a nicer bike for race day. While it's normally important to train on the bike you're planning to race on, if you have a pretty progressive bike shop in the area, you may be able to rent a good-quality bike for race day. Make sure to take it for a test ride and have them double-check everything on the bike. Renting is also a good option if you're traveling to a race. The big downside of renting a bike is it'll be an unfamiliar piece of equipment and feel a heck of a lot different from the one you've been training on.

At the end of the day, the most important thing is to make sure your bike is dependable. You don't want to train for a race only to have your bike break down on you. Game over. Make sure it fits your size, and whether it's a mountain bike, a commuter or your 15-year-old 10-speed, it'll suffice.

BIKE ACCESSORIES

The most important safety gear worn during a triathlon is a **bike helmet**. In fact, you won't be allowed to mount your bike until you clip yours on coming out of transition.

Make sure it fits well and stays in place on your head; a helmet should never slide around or it'll do you no good in an accident if it moves into an improper position during impact. It's a very good idea to replace your helmet often, as the space-age foam that keeps your brain bucket safe hardens over time and will provide less protection in a crash. Check out the manufacturer's website for fit and replacement guidelines.

Make sure you practice how to put on your helmet quickly; the transition from swimming to biking is complicated enough, and you don't want to get hung up by fighting with your helmet strap.

To clip or not to clip, is that really a question? At some point in your career, you'll have to make the decision to purchase special **bike shoes and pedals** that mate together and clip in to give you an advantage pedaling the bike, rather than using a "basket"-style pedal that allows you to wear your running shoes during the ride. As a beginner, that decision is probably at least a few races away. While you do have an advantage using a bike shoe due to its ability to transfer power more efficiently with each stroke of the cranks, for the short bike distance of a sprint, a newbie triathlete can easily get by without making that investment. (Yet.)

There are a few different types of **bike bags** that you'll need. An under-seat bag is a necessity; use it to hold extra tubes and tools to repair a flat. A "bento" bag for the top of the frame that attaches just behind the stem is a must-have if you'll be eating any solid foods or gels during a race.

SWIMMING GEAR

You'll need to pick up a pair of swim **goggles**, and a $10 pair from your local sports shop will work just fine. The most important thing is that they fit your face properly and don't leak. Do not wait until the race to try on new goggles; you should already have swum with them and adjusted them prior to the race.

Score! You can keep your wallet in your pocket for **swim caps**. They'll give them out at the event and are covered by your entry fee.

If the race is wetsuit-legal, then you should seriously consider using one. If you're not an extremely strong and fast swimmer, the advantage of using a **wetsuit** is immeasurable. A proper triathlon wetsuit will make you much more buoyant and able to conserve energy during the swim. With the wetsuit you can worry a lot less about staying afloat, and you'll also have less drag through the water. Elite triathletes regularly swim a 1500-meter distance event 90 seconds quicker with wetsuits on.

A wetsuit will take a decent amount of abuse during a race, so for your first wetsuit, you shouldn't go too crazy; there are plenty of entry-level triathlon wetsuits for less than $200, and if you shop during the off-season you'll find some great deals. If you're not ready to buy just yet, look to local triathlon shops in your area or even online for triathlon wetsuit rentals. A triathlon wetsuit is designed specifically for what you're trying to use it for, and any other wetsuits are not. Don't try to wear a cheap surf or scuba suit—it's a recipe for disaster.

When choosing your triathlon wetsuit, look at the size chart, and if you're between sizes, always size one up. The most competitive racers tend to sacrifice comfort and wear their suits uncomfortably tight, while the weekend warriors tend to err on the side of comfort and use a slightly larger suit. Do make sure you can pull it up as high as possible to provide full range of arm motion. Also, be sure that the zipper on your triathlon wetsuit is on your back, not running down the front of your torso. This happens at every triathlon.

One of the most vital purchases that can be made along with a wetsuit is an **anti-chafe skin-lubricant product** like Body Glide, Naked Surf or Aquaphor. Apply it liberally around your neck every time you wear your wetsuit in races or training to prevent the all-too-common wetsuit rash. These products are also really effective to help you remove your wetsuit. Coat the front and back of your calves before you slip the suit on and it'll slide off much more easily when you go to remove it.

RUNNING GEAR

It's very important to have a comfortable pair of **running shoes** that provides the support and cushioning you'll need. If the shoes are prone to giving you blisters in training, you should invest in a new pair. Just make sure you break them in before the race. If you're new to buying shoes, we highly recommend stopping by a full-service shoe store with knowledgeable staff who can examine your gait on a treadmill and help you pick the proper shoe. Many experienced triathletes opt for shoes with a built-in

sock liner with minimal seams to prevent blisters even when they're not wearing socks. A lot of high-end running shoes feature this option. Try as many as it takes to get the right fit. Be prepared to spend around a hundred dollars for the right shoes; comfortable running shoes are worth every penny.

CLOTHING & ACCESSORIES

You may not have the most high-tech, streamlined triathlon bike, but being as aerodynamic as possible is still very important. Any clothing that catches the wind will cause significant drag and make you work much harder during the entire bike leg. Yes, this is the reason folks wear some ridiculously tight-fitting outfits; otherwise it's a "drag" out on the bike course. And remember, the more stuff you have on, the more time it will take to mess around with it in transition. Make sure you have what you need without going overboard on unnecessary layers, gadgets and gizmos. Make sure to read through the "Triathlon Race-Day Checklist" (page 35).

Tri Suit / Swim Suit Tri suits are the most popular garb, and they can be an all-in-one jumpsuit or two pieces consisting of a top and bottom. This gear is designed to be worn through the entire race: under the wetsuit during the swim and by itself on the bike and run. There are so many other things to think about during a triathlon, and wearing a tri suit allows you to cross "attire" off your

TRIATHLON RACE-DAY CHECKLIST

See page 135 for a tear-out version or download a printable version of this list at www.7weekstofitness.com.

PRE-/POST-RACE GEAR
- ❑ Warm Clothes/Jacket
- ❑ Sandals
- ❑ Cap/Visor
- ❑ Change of Clothes
- ❑ Pre-/Post-Race Nutrition

SWIM
- ❑ Swimsuit/Wetsuit
- ❑ Goggles

BIKE
- ❑ Bike (tuned, tires inflated)
- ❑ Bike Shoes
- ❑ Helmet
- ❑ Water Bottles
- ❑ On-Bike Nutrition (energy gels, bars)
- ❑ Sunglasses

RUN
- ❑ Shoes
- ❑ Socks (if necessary)
- ❑ Race Belt with Number
- ❑ Run Nutrition (energy gels, bars)

TRANSITION
- ❑ Sunscreen
- ❑ Anti-Chafe/Skin Lubricant
- ❑ Water Bottle
- ❑ Towel
- ❑ Shorts (if necessary)
- ❑ Shirt (if necessary)

list. For the most part, they're tight yet comfortable. The wind-cheating design is most certainly body-hugging and engineered for the specific task at hand: racing in a triathlon. With the built-in pockets for holding nutrition on the bike and run as well as the chamois/padding in the groin for bike comfort, they do the job extremely well.

Not ready for body-hugging Lycra? Start with a swim suit, add bike shorts with a race singlet or bike jersey in transition 1, and swap the bike shorts for running shorts at transition 2. Bear in mind that at most short course events, there's usually no modesty tent and no nudity is allowed in transition; the swimsuit you started the day with will be your bottom layer until the finish line.

Socks Socks are a personal choice. If you're prone to blisters, then they're a good idea. If you can get by without them you'll save yourself some time fighting with getting them on with wet and dirty feet. If you're wearing bike shoes that fit properly, you most likely will not need socks, as your feet should not be moving around inside the shoes while you pedal. Running shoes with sock liners are a popular choice for those looking to get through the run without having to put socks on. Make sure you practice running with and without socks in training. The last thing you want is to try something new on race day and end up limping through the final miles with a painful blister. A non-chafe product like Body Glide can also be applied to your feet if you're prone to blisters and can help a great deal.

Race Belt You're required to wear your race number during the run at all events, and sometimes even on the bike. Picking up a race belt for as little as $5 is a better option than pinning a number on your race attire, and you get to avoid those pesky snags and holes that can ruin your expensive shirts. Simply attach your number to the belt and clip it on in transition before you head out for the bike or run.

Sun Protection A visor or hat is a great idea on the run in sunny conditions, as is applying some waterproof sunscreen to all the areas that'll be exposed on the bike and run before you get into your wetsuit. Re-applying spray-on sunscreen before the run can also be smart in longer events. Some ultra distance events even have designated volunteers to slather sunscreen on you before you head out to the run!

The Event

Once you've made it to race day, there are only about a billion things to remember. Luckily, we included a checklist on page 35 to help you remember most items. Make a few copies, or it may look a bit strange walking around transition with this book in your hands—although it may be great for us!

BEFORE THE RACE

Many larger events hold a race expo/packet pickup the day before a race, and often those events will let you drop your bike off early. Don't worry, they hire security guards to watch the bikes overnight. Events of this type are probably very organized and have pre-determined spots in transition for each athlete's bike based on their race number. If that's the case, you simply need to find your designated spot in transition and drop your bike off. This makes for less confusion on race-day morning and even during the race—it's easier to find your spot if you follow the numbers!

Events that don't have a numbering system on the bike racks can be a bit of a free-for-all, with bikes getting crammed in at all times on race morning. If this is the case, get there early and claim a spot that's easy to get to from the transition entrances and exits, then rack your bike and lay out your gear. If it's crowded and busy, there's a good chance you'll get your bike and gear shoved around a little bit as everyone tries to find space. Keep an even temper, remember that there's a good chance most other athletes are as excited and nervous as you are, and try to compromise for the good of all racers.

On race morning, eat a light breakfast a couple hours before the start. This meal should be similar to those you've had during training and not something heavy that will sit in your stomach. Experiment with different meals in training so you know what will provide you energy but not send you to the Porta-Potties. Arrive at the race early; if you've racked your bike the night before, find it and lay out your stuff. If you have to rack your bike in the morning, you'll probably be lugging a lot of gear while pushing a bike. Your wetsuit, goggles, nutrition and all the gear on your checklist should be in a backpack so you're not performing a juggling act from the parking lot to transition.

SETTING UP YOUR TRANSITION GEAR

There's usually one central transition area where you'll rack your bike and keep your gear. Only athletes are

> Most races have specific rules regarding wearing ear buds and impose penalties if you're caught wearing them. Even if you use them in training, leave them home on race day—and don't even think about donning them during the bike leg!

permitted inside the transition area, so you'll have to lug all of your stuff in and set up by yourself. Set up your gear in a small area under your bike; a bath towel folded in half is usually about the amount of personal space you have on the ground below your bike. Lay out the gear you'll need in the order you'll use it:

- Hang your wetsuit over your bike; you'll put that on after you're done with body marking and made any necessary trips to the Porta-Potties.

- Wear your swim goggles around your neck; you can't misplace them there. If you keep them in your hands you'll invariably lose them. Heed this warning.

- Place your bike gear down first on the towel, followed by your running gear.

- Don't forget your sunglasses; place them in your bike helmet.

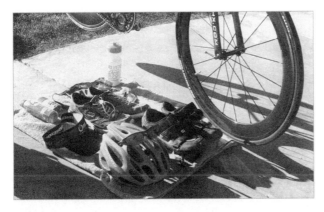

- Lay out any nutrition or hydration you'll want in transition or to take with you on the run. Your bike should have bottle holders; make sure you bring an appropriate amount of hydration for the distance and conditions.

- Once you get your bike racked and gear set, find the volunteers walking around transition with markers to write your race number on your arms and your age on your calf before you put on your wetsuit. This is called "body marking," and there are usually lines of athletes waiting to get marked.

- Return to your spot and re-check your gear; mentally plan how you'll execute your transitions.

- Apply waterproof sunscreen to all areas that'll be exposed to sun during the bike and run.

- Apply anti-chafe to the area around your neck where the wetsuit will rub, as well as any other region where your skin will be rubbed. Most products like Body Glide, Aquaphor and Naked Surf are waterproof and one application is good for the entire race.

- Listen for announcements from race organizers regarding start times, and put on your wetsuit before walking toward the water.

- Help your neighbor pull up their wetsuit zipper and they'll return the favor.

- Make sure you remember the swim cap that came in your race packet; you'll usually line up before the swim based on age groups and corresponding swim cap colors.

THE RACE: GETTING THROUGH THE LEGS

Most races start in "waves" of athletes divided by age group with 3 to 5 minutes between wave starts, reducing the number of athletes starting together in the water. However, all Ironman triathlons are a mass start with all the competitors starting together in the water.

It's up to you where you position yourself in the packs of swimmers in the water. Strong swimmers are encouraged to position themselves toward the front of the wave for a less-crowded path through the water, while weaker swimmers should stay near the back and outer edges of the wave to avoid possibly being swum over. There's plenty of water safety, and if you get tired, disoriented or scared, you can hang onto a kayak, surfboard or lifeguard for as long as you want without being disqualified. However, bear in mind that you also may not advance your position on the course while holding onto a ledge, kayak or any other object.

Your initial reaction at the starter's gun may be to swim as hard as you can. Don't do it! Take it easy until you find your pace and develop a comfortable stroke and breathing pattern. It's quite common to count the rhythm of your strokes, kicks and breathing to keep them smooth and even. It's important that you pace yourself early in the swim; once you hit your rhythm you'll speed up.

After exiting the water, remove your goggles, unzip your wetsuit and pull it over your shoulders down to your waist as you hustle toward your bike in transition. There should be volunteers showing you the way, as well as a Swim In sign. Now it's up to you to locate your bike. Remove your wetsuit fully and get into your bike gear, making sure to strap on your helmet and run your bike to the Bike Out sign. Do not mount your bike until after the "Mount Here" line. If it's crowded at the mount line, you can jog your bike up a little farther while trying to stay out of other athletes' ways.

Head out on the bike course and be aware of other cyclists around you. It's normally congested in the first few miles, so be careful not to clip the wheels of cyclists in front of you. For the most part, if you're in a pack, you shouldn't make any drastic moves unless you have the clear space to accelerate and pass slower riders. In bunched-up situations like this, officials will usually not penalize someone for drafting, but when the opportunity arises to spread out, make sure you do. Remember to stay to the right unless passing and to stay about three bike lengths behind the rider in front of you. When drinking from your water bottle, make sure you have some flat, straight road ahead of you and no cyclists too close so you don't cause any accidents while taking a drink.

After finishing the bike course, get off your bike at the Unmount Here line and run your bike back to your original rack position. Change into your running gear, apply sunscreen if needed, clip on your race belt and run to the Run Out sign.

Pace yourself during the run; with all the adrenaline coursing through your veins it's easy to push too hard too soon. Find an even pace that you can maintain and tick off the miles step by step.

Most races will have race photographers throughout the event, but the best opportunity for a photo to remember is during the run—especially at the finish line. No matter how tired you may be, once you spot the photographer, do your best to make it look like you're having the time of your life (well, you are, right?).

Triathlon Rules

There are the general rules that govern all triathlons sanctioned by organizations such as USAT, and then there are race-specific rules. It's your responsibility to be aware of all the rules for your event. Read through the event rules on the website and attend pre-race meetings to find out important information like whether the event allows wetsuits for the swim or earphones on the run, as well as specific guidelines for transition entrances, exits, and bike mounts. "I didn't know" is not an acceptable excuse (is it ever?), so it's up to you to be knowledgeable and prepared when you show up to race.

The basic rules for a triathlon:

- You may not use any motorized propulsion during the swim, bike or run. Flippers, flotation devices and personal watercraft are entirely illegal.

- Athletes may not receive any outside help other than that of race volunteers at designated aid stations or on-course bike repair technicians. Praying to your deity of choice to get you through the swim is perfectly acceptable.

- Bicycle helmets must be worn before mounting the bike when leaving transition onto the bike leg and may not be removed until after dismounting the bike when returning to transition. Make sure to remove your bike helmet before the run. Seriously, it happens more than you might think.

- When on the bike, a cyclist must stay to the right of the course when not passing and allow other competitors to pass on the left. A violation of this is considered "blocking." (See "Hell on Wheels: The Bike Course" on page 29.)

- In almost all triathlons, drafting is illegal. Cyclists must maintain approximately three bike lengths (7 meters) distance from the cyclist in front of them, and if within that distance, must complete a pass of the forward cyclist within 15 seconds or drop back out of the drafting zone. For more on drafting, see page 131.

- Entry and exit of transition must be done via the proper route in the proper sequence. In events where timing chips are involved, going into or out of transition through the wrong gate may result in disqualification and, even worse, public humiliation. Just follow the big signs and the volunteers and you should be A-OK.

- Thank your volunteers, be helpful and respectful of other athletes, and remember to tip your waitresses. Seriously, triathlons can be extremely stressful and occasionally you'll meet some rude, self-absorbed people; just make sure you're not one of them.

Progressing in Races

Most mountain climbers don't start out by scaling Mount Everest, and in triathlons newbies should not attempt to start out at an ultra distance. It's highly recommended that your first few triathlons be a sprint distance, and then you can progress to longer distances after you've learned more about the sport and improved as a multisport athlete. If your goal is to progress to a long course or even an ultra distance, here's an example of a reasonable race progression:

- Compete in sprint distance triathlons for about three months and gain experience, confidence and skill.

- Between races, extend your distances in each discipline, shooting for the swim, bike and run duration of your next target event.

- Enter a 10k running race before moving up to an Olympic or mid-distance event to see how you can handle running double the distance of sprints during a competitive event.

- After competing in mid-distance triathlons for another one to three months, sign up for a half marathon and test your running ability at the 13.1-mile distance.

- If you're consistent with adding distance and quality workouts to your training over the next one to three months, you should be ready to compete in a long-distance triathlon.

Moving up to an ultra distance triathlon is a huge leap from long-distance and requires a great deal of training. Most triathletes will train hard for an ultra that's 3 to 6 months away by drastically increasing their training volume. This training will often include two workouts a day and extremely long-distance runs and bike rides on weekends.

Prior to signing up for an ultra distance, it's a good idea to have at least 1 or 2 marathons under your belt and routinely bike 80 to 100 miles.

Taking It to the Next Level

Say that one day you're out playing tennis at the local park and you hit a ball about two city blocks over the fence in the wrong direction. Just when you decide to go retrieve your wayward ball, John McEnroe walks through the fence holding it in his hand.

"You know," he says, "I can see you're training hard to get better at tennis. Why don't I write down 35 or so of my personal secret tips and techniques for you? Better yet, why don't I give you an easy-to-follow training plan to make you a better tennis player while I'm at it?"

That sort of thing happens all the time, right? Well, it does right here in this book. We've put together 35 tips that Lewis has learned over the last decade as a professional triathlete to make you a faster, more efficient racer. Pick the ones that match your weaknesses and get training!

IMPROVE YOUR TRANSITIONS

1 Focus on T1 and T2 as being the fourth and fifth disciplines of your triathlon. This is not a time to rest, but a time to focus on sheer speed and not waste time. Too many people don't keep the same intensity during transition as they do during the swim, bike and run. Sometimes it seems that transitions should perhaps be at an elevated intensity, as minimal mistakes can cost you crucial seconds.

2 Always look for a good spot! Before the race, know where you'll run in from the swim, come in from your bike and run out for your run. If the transition spots aren't assigned by race number, arrive early and select the best spot. This usually means you'll travel the least distance in the transition area, have the most room, and won't be impeded by others. Use your best judgment and try to imagine what the area will look like during the race.

3 When setting up, identify your transition spot by a tree or an immobile landmark of some kind. Remember that things will look different when the area is emptier during the race. Find something that's simple but will help you locate your bike or running gear. Note that the other competitors' equipment will not be there to key off of when you arrive. Some people even tie a balloon to their spot; if it's allowed at your particular race, why not?

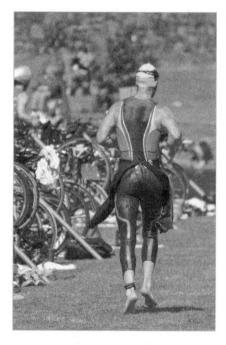

4 Place all your running gear farther back under your bike in the transition rack, and make sure it's organized. Everything can get tossed about by you and your transition-mates during T1, and pushing your run gear farther under the rack helps ensure that it'll be there when you're rushing through T2. Remember that what seems easy and logical at rest sometimes becomes very difficult when very fatigued!

GET SMOOTHER IN THE TRANSITIONS, BABY!

Transitions are often overlooked as an area to improve in triathlon, but getting them down is key. The clock is always running, and T1 and T2 can make or break a race at the higher levels. To become faster and more efficient, practice completing perfect transitions over and over in training, including in an extremely fatigued state.

To practice, set up a transition area near the swimming pool, mimicking as close to race-day conditions as you can. Get into your tri suit or swimming gear and lay out your transition with everything you would have in a race: your number belt, nutrition, helmet, sunglasses, etc. Warm up in the pool, do a 100-meter nearly-all-out swim, then exit the pool and run to your mock transition. Put on your bike gear and run the bike about 20 yards before mounting. Ride hard for 1 mile, return back to transition, and change into your run gear. Run hard for 1 mile, return back to the transition, and assess your mistakes. Rearrange your gear and do the drill again while trying to correct any area that needs improvement. After you've made a few attempts and feel pretty efficient, start timing yourself and see if you can keep improving. Repeat 5 or even 10 or more times for a great workout!

5 Always place a distinctive towel on the ground where you plan to put on your running shoes in T2. Not only does the towel feel good on your feet, but it dries and cleans them too. Also, it's a good way to quickly locate precisely where your spot is in your row, which can sometimes be difficult when most of the bikes are still out on the course!

6 Use Body Glide around your wrists and ankles so you can take your wetsuit off more quickly and it won't stick to your skin. When exiting the water after the swim and running to transition, strip your wetsuit down to your waist. By the time you get to your bike, you'll only have to yank it off your legs.

7 Position your bike on the rack so it's heading in the direction you want to exit transition. When possible, most pros rack their bikes by the saddle rather than the handlebars as it allows the bike to already be rolling forward without the need of turning it around in the transition area. This may seem like a small detail, but if it's crowded during T1, you'll be glad you did it this way—every second counts.

8 Use tri-specific shoes and have them already clipped into the pedals. Exit transition without your shoes on, pedal up to speed with your feet on top of your shoes and then put them on while already at race speed. Please note that this takes an incredible amount of dexterity and practice, and is not recommended to anyone who doesn't have 100 percent confidence that they can complete the task on race day.

9 Take note of the race topography immediately out of transition on the bike ride and adjust your plan accordingly. Is there a steep hill? You may want to put your shoes on before getting on your bike. Is there a moderate hill? You may leave your shoes on your bike, but you'll want to be in the small chain ring or an easier gear so you have less trouble getting up to speed.

10 Put on your arm warmers/coolers and sunglasses while you're on the bike. A little piece of tape can keep your sunglasses in place on your handlebars until you're ready; don't try to run out of transition with anything other than your bike in your hands. Like tip #8, this takes some practice to perform comfortably.

11 Leaving transition for the bike leg can often be very crowded and quite dangerous. In this case, try to hold your position and stay out of trouble until you get out onto a main road, where passing and going fast are a little safer. This may not seem like a tip to go faster, but if you clip another rider leaving transition your day may be over before the bike leg even begins.

12 Some triathletes save lots of time in transition by not having to tie their running shoes. Use a product like "lace locks" or elastic laces, which allows you to slide your shoes on and take off running without spending time tying the shoes. These can save more than 30 seconds of precious time over someone using conventional laces.

13 Forgo socks! I generally don't wear socks for sprint or middle-distance triathlons. With proper-fitting bike shoes, your feet should not slide around and cause friction or discomfort. When the run distance is longer than 10k, I wear socks as they can help prevent blisters and foot discomfort.

MASTER THE SWIM

14 Do some intensity work EVERY time you swim. Swimming isn't like cycling and running; because it's low-impact, you can do some hard stuff every time out. This doesn't mean an all-out effort every minute you're in the pool, but put in some good, hard intervals every time you're training.

15 Join a masters swim team. "Masters" is kind of misleading and basically just means "adult swim club." Masters workouts are almost always on the clock using swim intervals. It's vital that you swim in this manner not only to improve, but to realize when you're improving. Swimmers and triathletes usually don't get why masters swimming will make them so much better until they do it, so just do it!

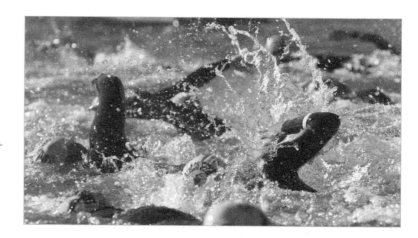

16 Start a swim-specific weights program. This will mostly look like a basic lifting program for the core, upper body and lower body. If you have any weaknesses in muscle strength, this could help your swimming significantly. See "Cross-Training for Triathlon Success" on page 90.

17 Drill drill drill. There are a great number of swim drills to focus on, but a good rule of thumb is if you feel like you struggle with a certain drill, you probably need that drill the most. Incorporate drilling into your swim every time you get in the water.

18 Practice like you race: open water. Go out and do an open-water swim once a week, and at least once a month. Most triathlons take place in open bodies of water, and swimming in them is usually significantly different from swimming in a pool. There's a basic "learning curve" that happens over time, but even the most seasoned swimmer can benefit from practicing in the open water. It's a good way to practice swimming in your wetsuit, treading water as you would at the start and swimming without the rest of the wall every few strokes. Open-water swimming will force you to practice spotting as well. If there's any chop, swimming in rough waters can be tricky without proper experience. Be ready for race day!

19 To prevent goggle fog, use baby shampoo. Rinse your goggles with a little baby shampoo before you head to the race. It drastically reduces fog buildup on your goggles. An even simpler solution is saliva right before you swim—to each their own!

20 Swim twice a day. No, not every day, but sometimes it's good to force yourself into swimming twice. You'll be amazed at the "feel" you have for the water the more you do this.

21 Many top triathletes do a "swim focus" in the off-season. Because swimming is so low-impact and fairly time efficient for someone who has swimming as their weakness, it's often a good idea to take November or December and swim as your main form of exercise. Sometimes athletes can make a big jump in ability, and it stays with them even when cycling and running are added to their training programs later. A couple notes of caution: If you do this, return to running and cycling slowly and cautiously—it's easy to get injured from too much too soon. Also, if your shoulders start to hurt from all the yards in the pool, be sure to ice them regularly. A good rule of thumb is if you feel a "pinch" in your shoulder, stop immediately; it's probably an injury. If your shoulders just "ache," it's probably just overuse and, though not perfectly comfortable, it's probably something that won't affect you long-term.

22 The most common problem for new swimmers, especially men, is body position. If your legs, hips and shoulders aren't right near the surface of the water,

THREE TOP TIPS TO IMPROVE YOUR SWIM TIME

Frank Sole, a swim coach and the owner of Sole Swim Solutions in Scottsdale, Arizona, helps pros and age-groupers alike train for their best triathlon swim. According to Frank, swimming is relatively simple: the ability to get from point A to point B in the most efficient way possible. Efficient swimming is 90% technique and 10% strength; the fastest swimmers follow the "Three Bs" below to cut through the water and expend as little energy as possible while covering the greatest possible distance.

1. BALANCE—In order to move through the water more easily, your body needs to be as balanced and streamlined as possible. Developing proper frontal and horizontal balance in the water takes time to master, but the benefits far outweigh the effort. For example, swimming with hips low in the water and head high creates drag, which creates resistance that robs you of momentum while sapping your energy. This brings us to the next B...

2. BODY POSITIONING—An effective swim stroke starts at the hips and moves outward toward the hands and legs, never the other way around. This helps to ensure balanced hip rotation from side to side. I remind my athletes that this "hip-first" body positioning helps create balance and make them more efficient with each rotation and stroke. Proper body position helps to minimize bilateral imbalances that lead to inefficient swimming.

3. BIOMECHANICS—The final "B" brings the first two together: The mechanics of swimming become radically easier when you master balance and body positioning; then you can add techniques. Some very effective ways to improve your biomechanics are: front-quadrant swimming, or catching the water in front of your body as early as possible; utilizing your hand along with your forearm as a paddle in a smooth stroke, and not dragging it back toward your body like a piston; maintaining a tight, compact kick that starts at the hips with minimal bending of the knees and feet pointing behind you like you're trying to touch the back wall with your toes.

then you're figuratively swimming uphill! People tend not to understand just how much pressure you need to push down with your chest to get into proper body position. Good swimmers do this naturally, as they've done it for so long they don't even realize it. Poor swimmers have to kick very hard just to keep their legs up, and they tire very quickly. A great way to improve this serious swimming flaw is to do 25s or 50s with your feet tied together with an elastic band, allowing for a slight bit of foot movement but not a traditional kick. With a road bicycle tube, you can make about three bands by cutting the tube into three pieces and tying each piece into three loops. Put the band around your ankles and try to swim down the

pool. (With a lifeguard on duty, of course!) Push down with your upper body until you're able to comfortably swim greater distances with the "band" around your ankles. When you take it off, your kick will now be for propulsive purposes rather than used to just keep your legs up. You won't believe how good it feels to swim once you've learned proper body position and balance!

23 Kick less! You'll find that very good swimmers, especially distance swimmers, have a very light and loose kick. Their kick is mainly for balance and timing, not for speed. The legs contain big muscles, and they're not nearly as powerful as the upper body for swimming.

Overusing their legs causes a swimmer to fatigue quickly, and usually results in significantly less speed. The next time you're tired during a longer swim, focus on a subtler and more relaxed kick. This will usually bring your heart rate down with very little or no reduced speed.

BLAZING PEDALS: GETTING SPEEDIER ON THE BIKE

24 Take a good look at what the top pros ride. Many of them ride the bikes they're paid to, but most ride what they think will allow them to do their best, especially at the pointy end of the field. Look at their helmets, bike setups, water bottles, wheels and whatever else you want when you wonder, "What's the fastest?" They've done all the research for their rig, and you can see it on display in transition. It's a heck of a lot cheaper than visiting a wind tunnel!

25 Do one-legged drills! I usually do these on a trainer, but you can also do them outdoors riding on a flat road with little traffic. Pedal with one leg on the pedal, the other out behind you or off to the side, in a medium-hard gear for 40 pedal strokes, then switch to the other leg and repeat. While you're doing these drills attempt to pedal with strokes and try not to let the chain slack at all; there should be smooth resistance for the whole 360 degrees of the pedal stroke. This will help you become more efficient and get rid of that "dead-spot" in your pedal stroke that many cyclists have.

26 Buy speed! Equipment choices, though often very expensive, can make you significantly faster. Once you're in very good shape, have optimized your cycling position, and feel like you've hit an improvement plateau, you can always buy something to make you faster; it's all about how much you're willing to spend. Here are some of the best options to buy speed by making yourself or the bike more aerodynamic (time savings over 40k time trial in parentheses): body-hugging tri suit (about 2:15 vs. shorts and T-shirt); aero bars (about 2:00 vs. standard handlebars); aero helmet (about 1:10 vs. standard helmet); front aero wheel (about :45 vs. aluminum rims); rear disc wheel (about :30 vs. aluminum rims); shoe covers (about :30 vs. none); aerodynamic triathlon frame (about :20 vs. standard triathlon frame).

Cost-wise, clip-on aero bars may be the best bang for your buck at less than $75, followed by a relatively high-end, wind-cheating tri suit at $250 and up. The more you progress as a triathlete, the more you'll seek out tips, techniques and gear to trim valuable minutes and seconds off your finishing time. Unfortunately, it doesn't come cheap!

27 Train on different bikes. A while back there was a study that found that of all types of cyclists (road, mountain, track, tri-riders), the most efficient pedal strokes were consistently those of mountain bikers. Why? Because when riding up incredibly steep hills where they struggle to maintain traction and not fall backward, a perfectly smooth pedal stroke is key to continued motion. This is something good mountain bikers develop over time by, you guessed it, mountain biking. It's no secret that the top triathlon cyclists often train on road bikes and do road races too, even though the position on the bike is significantly different. Get into various types of cycling to improve your bike speed overall. It takes time, and gains are sometimes not realized right away, but it's a good way to ensure you're doing your best to get faster.

28 Sign up for a bike race. This may sound a little dangerous and be way out of your comfort zone, but that's exactly why you should do it. Bike racing, even time trials (where the cyclist rides alone against the clock), are very different from multisport events and allow you to focus on one sport for that particular period of time. In mass-start events like criteriums and road races, tactics also play an important role in the dynamic and outcome of the event, adding another huge component to your understanding of the sport. This also makes it fun, and can be a challenge to do with other triathletes or cyclists and build camaraderie among your peers.

29 Inflate your tires to 115 psi or their allowable max! You can usually find this number on the sidewall of your tires. Too many people regularly ride and even race with soft tires. In most conditions, barring rain and very bumpy conditions, a little more inflation can make you significantly faster. It's not a bad idea to check your tire pressure with an accurate pump before each ride.

30 Clean and lubricate your bicycle chain, then clean it again. There's an amazing amount of energy a cyclist can lose in their chain if it's not clean and properly lubricated. There are many forms of chain lube, like White Lightning and Tri-Flow, that we highly recommend. The key is that your chain is very clean, and then after you apply the lubrication, you wipe the excess lube off the chain to keep grime from accumulating during that ride. I've seen people pick up a half mile per hour just by cleaning and lubricating their bike chain!

31 Ride an indoor trainer or rollers. Indoor trainers can improve your riding because they allow you to focus on nothing but the resistance from the trainer, as you aren't moving and there are no hazards to worry about. You can measure your power, heart rate and cadence and see how your body responds. Rollers, a form of trainer where you ride on drums without your bike locked in, can be very good for your pedal stroke and cycling balance. They also work well to ward off boredom during long indoor sessions. If you're riding hard, or long, indoors, you should keep the environment cool and have a fan on you as it's very easy to overheat. Also, change your wet bike shorts often to prevent blisters in some rather uncomfortable areas.

ON THE RUN

32 Run more frequently! There are many triathletes who believe in 30- or 90-day challenges where they try to run a set distance every day over a set period of time, barring injury. Frequency in running is key, as the more you run, the more your body learns an efficient stride and becomes comfortable under that form of exertion. Most running coaches believe triathletes tend to not run enough overall. Intervals, speed work and track workouts are great options to get more quality runs into your routine. Be aware that an increase in running is a significant increase in the chance of an overuse injury. Be very careful and stop at the first sign of pain—don't push through it. Also consider running on softer surfaces like grass, trail or even the treadmill as they should lower your risk of injury under increasing workload.

> Hands down, the best way to understand a race course is to train on it. Go for a swim in the lake, ride the bike route and put some miles in on the run course. Even if you do it on separate days, you'll have some familiarity of the course—and the upper-hand on your competition.
> —Mark H. Wilson, Race Director of HITS Triathlon Series

33 Catch overuse injuries before they become chronic. In contact sports, usually the most serious injuries come on rapidly, usually through a hard collision or a quick movement, and in a split second the damage is done. In endurance sports, like triathlon, we more often get what are called "overuse" injuries. These occur due to stress over time and usually there are precursors to the major injury. As we become more experienced, and more careful, we can learn how to identify those little aches and pains prior to them becoming more serious. Not every ache or niggle will become a major injury, but some will, and it's always good to err on the side of caution. RICE therapy is a good start (Rest, Ice, Compression, Elevation), as is seeing a sports therapist whom you trust. Common triathlon injuries are shoulder tendinitis (biceps, or rotator cuff), ITB (iliotibial band) syndrome, Achilles tendinitis, hip labrum issues, sacroiliac joint pain, patellar tendinitis, plantar fasciitis and many more. It's important to be cautious and get on these injuries before they become chronic!

34 Use compression for recovery. Compression socks and tights have become very popular in the running and triathlon community. Look for some tight yet comfortable compression wear to put on after hard workouts, and see if it aids your recovery. Some people swear by it, and others think it doesn't work for them—to each their own. You never know if you don't try! Relatively new to the market are compression boots, which work like a deep massage on the legs. Many top athletes are now using them, and while they're expensive they can help speed up recovery time. If you can't afford

LEWIS ELLIOT—GOING PRO

When I was a kid, my dad and I would set up mini triathlons and compete against each other, but once I watched Mark Allen and Dave Scott battle to the end in the 1989 "Iron War" as a nine year old, I was 100 percent captivated by the sport of triathlon. However, I was a poor swimmer and couldn't make the time commitment to the local swim team, so my mom persuaded me to focus on cycling or running—I chose cycling. By age 15 I was a successful Category 1 rider racing with some of the most elite cyclists in the U.S., and I was regularly winning races around Florida. When my friends were getting their driver's licenses, I was the Junior National Cycling Champion.

However, about the time I was becoming a serious threat on a bike, my world came crashing down. In 1996, my mother, who seemed perfectly healthy, was diagnosed with stage-4 breast cancer. In an instant, cycling was no longer my focus. My mother, a brave competitor in her own right, resiliently fought back against the cancer ravaging her body and encouraged me to continue pushing to be the best cyclist I could be.

From 1997 to 2000, I had the honor of being a member of the U.S. National Cycling Team, competing all over the world with teammates such as Dave Zabriskie, Danny Pate and Christian Vande Velde. But after a couple of years, I decided it was time to go back home. The following summer, I entered my first real triathlon, the Montana Big Sky State Games Sprint Tri. I had always been a quick runner and had developed a great deal of leg strength from cycling, but I was still a relatively miserable swimmer. After what seemed like an eternity in the water and a rough trip through my T1, I got on the bike course and made up a lot of time, moving up many places. I continued to close the gap on the run, and finished just three or four minutes behind Todd Struckman, the winner of the race, a pro triathlete who had also been victorious the three previous years. The instant I crossed the finish line, I knew I had found my sport, and that this would be my new passion.

A month later, I competed at the age-group Olympic Distance National Championships in Coeur d'Alene, Idaho. I struggled through the swim, but on the bike I rode the fastest split of the day. A solid 34-minute 10k later, I finished with an overall time of 2:02. A week later I submitted the paperwork for a "pro" card and, at 21 years old, after my second triathlon ever, my pro triathlon career began.

As a professional triathlete, the competition is often brutal, yet I'm extremely grateful to compete with top professional athletes like Tim DeBoom, Chris Lieto, Craig "Crowie" Alexander, Chris "Macca" McCormack and even Lance Armstrong. I continue to train and improve my craft, and in 2011 at Ford Ironman Arizona I set a PB (personal best) with a time of 8:38 for an Ironman event. I feel the passion for the sport of triathlon as strong as ever, and feel my best years of competition are still ahead.

to purchase them, some rehab or sports massage clinics have compression boots available for rental, which may be something to consider during your hardest training for a big event.

35 One final tip: Get over it. Good or bad, you need to learn to keep focusing on the goal ahead and not your recent achievements or failures. In order to excel in the sport of triathlon, you'll need to learn to get over quite a few bumps, bruises, injuries, setbacks, rude competitors, cranky officials, and your gear betraying you, your body betraying you, and more often than not your mind betraying you as well. A "perfect" race is like the Easter Bunny: No matter how much you believe in it, the simple reality is that it just doesn't exist. Even your PR (personal record) will always be less than perfect, and there's always something you could've done better. You'll surely have good races and bad races during your career; the key is to remember that even after setting a new personal best you haven't "figured it all out." At the next race you toe the starting line with everything to prove all over again. Your competitors don't care what you did last race, the course doesn't care about your new PR and there's no guaranteed positive outcome based on past successes. Get over it, and put out your best effort in order to yield the best result!

So You're Thinking about Going Pro?

Can you make a living racing triathlons? Do you think you have what it takes to be a pro?

With some natural ability and the desire to devote extensive time to each of the three disciplines, you may be ready to make the leap. Optimally, you should have some really positive results from recent events; possibly you were in the top three in one leg or even made the podium. Bear in mind that it requires a significant investment to equip yourself with pro-caliber gear and possibly hire a coach.

There are hundreds of pro triathletes and thousands, if not tens of thousands, who would like to make a living racing tris. It's a competitive business, like any profession with this much demand and relatively limited availability. There are a few people making a great living racing as a pro, but most professional triathletes are not making much money and usually have (or need) another means of income. Besides being a very fast triathlete, most successful pros are also well-spoken, consistent and excellent at marketing themselves. Anyone who hopes to be a pro one day should realistically assess their current level, their background in endurance sports and their financial position before deciding it's what they're going to pursue. Professional triathlon is all encompassing, and it's a huge commitment and a tough sport, but with success can be incredibly rewarding.

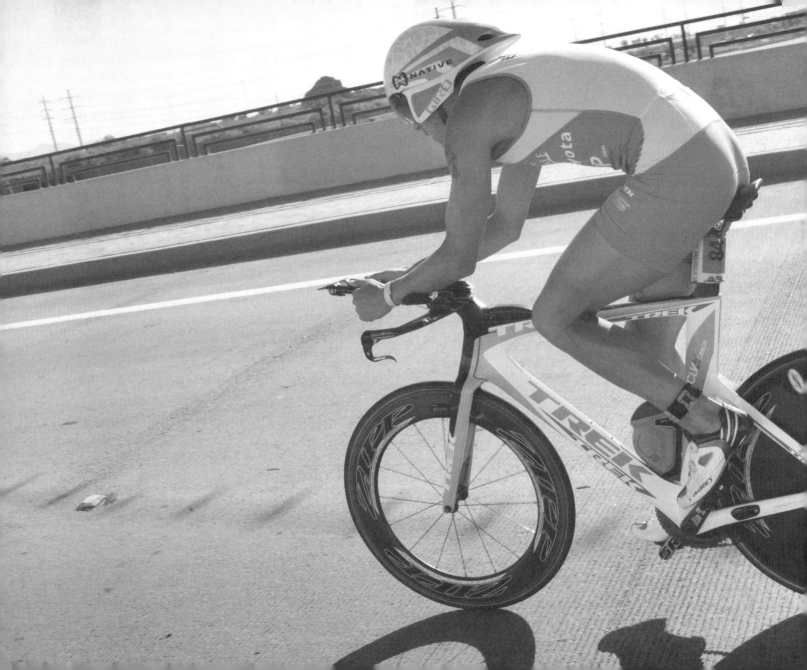

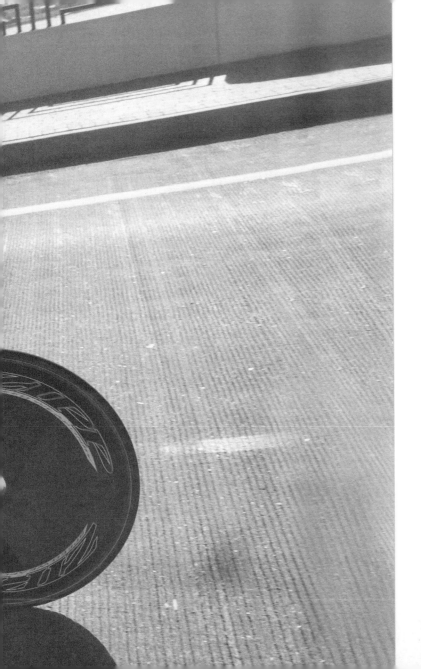

PART 2:
THE
PROGRAMS

7 Weeks to a Triathlon Programs

Your journey to becoming a triathlete starts with the Beginner Program, a 7-week immersion into the world of multisport training that features discipline-specific and "brick" workouts to prepare your mind and body for your first event. To help you keep track of the workouts, each week has a log entry where you can jot notes and reminders of your progress.

For the experienced triathlete, the Advanced Program begins on page 73 and provides a 7-week regimen to push your limits and boost your performance to amazing new levels. Even if you're not ready for the full "pro-caliber" workout, intermediate triathletes can add some of the Advanced drills into their own workouts to strengthen and improve as a multisport athlete.

Beginner Program

Are you ready to become a triathlete? We created this program for first-timers, relative beginners looking to improve by following a consistent program and even experienced triathletes who have taken some time off and want to get back into race shape.

This program should look particularly different than the ones you'll find in other publications, as it was specifically written as if we were right there next to you, speaking with you as a coach would. This flexible program gives beginner triathletes options while allowing them to learn and progress at their own rate.

When starting this program, it is imperative that you have a clean bill of health and are cleared by a doctor to participate in a taxing physical exercise program. You'll also need the necessary equipment to swim, bike and run (see "The Gear" starting on page 31). Last but not least, pick a race that's about 7 weeks away and sign up!

In order to jump right into this program, you should meet some minimum guidelines. You should be able to:

- Swim at least one length of a 25-yard pool without stopping

- Ride a bike about 5 miles

- Run or jog continuously for at least 3 minutes

Don't worry if you don't meet those requirements right off the bat—just use week 1 as your baseline for success. Follow the training plan as best as you can to progressively build up your swim, bike and run until you can complete the full week's program!

Reading the Beginner Charts

If you've never done a multisport-specific training regimen before, this program is a good indoctrination to the world of triathlon training. Each day will consist of swimming, biking, running or cross-training (or a combination of two or more). Each week has one off-day to rest.

Swim distances will be calculated by yards or lengths of the pool, so you may need some math to convert the workouts to the pool you're using. If you're lucky enough to be training in open water, a waterproof GPS watch may prove to be invaluable.

For repeats and duration like " 0x00," the first number is how many times you'll repeat the drill, and the second is the duration (distance or time). For example, "8x1 length" means you'll swim 1 length of the pool and repeat 8 times with the desired rest between sets; "3x3 minutes" or "3x3:00" should be read as 3 repeats of that drill for 3-minute durations each time.

When no specific amount of rest is given, the goal is to catch your breath and mentally prepare for the next set; :30 to 1:00 is average. You're training, not dilly-dallying.

"Race pace" refers to your goal pace for a sprint triathlon: a 500–700 meter swim, 12.4-mile bike and 3.1-mile run.

A "straight" swim means no stopping through the entire distance.

Week 1

DAY 1 Mon	**SWIM** 8x1 Length (beginning swimmer) OR 12x1 Length (proficient swimmer)

Triathlon starts with the swim, so that's how we'll kick off the training program. If you're a proficient swimmer, swim 300 yards today, or 12 lengths of a 25-yard pool. If you're brand-new to swimming, swim 8x1 length, resting at each end for a total of 200 yards. Take as much rest as you need after each length before continuing into your next. If you're new to swimming, see if there's someone at the pool who swims well and ask them to give you just two tips on how you could swim a little better. Efficient swimming is all about technique, so take all the help you can find!

DAY 2 Tue — **BIKE** 45- to 60-Minute Spin Class OR 30-Minute Exercise Bike

Spin class! Go to your local gym or YMCA and do a class. If you can't do that, get on an exercise bike and ride 30 minutes, attempting to work up a good sweat.

DAY 3 Wed — **RUN** 1-Mile Run

Do this on a treadmill or outside, or on a track if there's one nearby. If you can't run this far, then run for 1 minute and walk for 1 minute until you complete the mile.

DAY 4 Thu — **SWIM** 16x1 Lengths (beginning swimmer) OR 5x100 Yards (proficient swimmer)

For beginners, rest as needed after each length until you catch your breath, then go again. You can wear fins today if you have them. If you're a proficient swimmer, rest for 30 seconds after each 4 lengths.

NOTES: _____

DAY 5 Fri

REST
Did you read that correctly? That means you'll rest and recover with no strenuous physical activity in order to prepare for tomorrow!

DAY 6 Sat

BIKE/RUN BRICK   60-Minute Spin Class OR 45-Minute Bike Ride; 800-Meter Run
There is a chance your legs will feel like bricks after you've completed today's workout. Do a 60-minute spin class, or an easy 45 minutes on your exercise bike or bicycle, then run 800 meters straight. If you can't run the 800 meters, then run/walk it. Notice the feeling your legs have running directly after riding—it's tough! Make the transition as quickly as possible to the run. Have your running shoes out and ready, and don't take time to change clothes.

DAY 7 Sun

CROSS-TRAIN   1 Hour
Try to do 1 hour of a non-triathlon sport and work hard at it. If it goes more than 1 hour, that's OK! Go out and have fun! It's important to spend some time doing something other than tri training to keep your workouts exciting, but if you decide to absolutely have to swim/bike/run, split it up over an hour.

NOTES: _____

_____

_____

_____

_____

_____

_____

_____

_____

_____

NEWBIE TIP: Find out how long your local pool is; 20, 22.5 and 25 yards are fairly common, and it's often difficult to tell the difference. This will matter more and more as your distances increase, and you'll need to do some math to convert "300 yards" to fit your laps in a 22.5 yard pool.

Week 2

DAY 8 Mon

REST

This means COMPLETE rest...so enjoy it! Your body needs time to recover, heal and strengthen, and you probably need to do some laundry to have your gear ready for this week!

DAY 9 Tue

BIKE   45- to 60-Minute Bike Ride

Cycle harder than you did on Day 2 last week for 45–60 minutes. Push it—try to get a little out of breath. You can ride indoors, but outside is preferable because of the wind drag and terrain and temperature differences. Your triathlon will be outside and it's a great idea to train in similar conditions whenever possible.

DAY 10 Wed

RUN   1.5-Mile Run

Try to run the whole way; if you can't, run/walk/jog, but cover the distance!

DAY 11 Thu

SWIM   8x50 Yards (beginning swimmer) OR 12x50 Yards (proficient swimmer)

Try to go 8x50 yards in the pool. This is down and back, no stopping at the turn. After each 50 yards, rest 30 seconds, then go again. If you're a decent swimmer, go 12x50 and try to do them fairly hard, like your race pace for 400 meters.

NOTES: _____

_____

_____

_____

_____

_____

_____

_____

_____

_____

_____

_____

DAY 12 Fri

CROSS-TRAIN   Cross-Training Program A (page 92)

DAY 13 Sat

BIKE/RUN BRICK   60-Minute Bike Ride; 1-Mile Run
Bike for 1 hour and make sure at least 10 minutes is at a higher intensity, where talking is a little difficult because you're breathing quickly. Go from the bike to immediately putting on running shoes, and run 1 mile. Try to make the last 400 meters (.25 mile) a faster pace. If you can't run the whole mile, just run/walk it.

DAY 14 Sun

RUN/SWIM BRICK   3-Mile Run; 600-Yard Swim
Run 3 miles, the last mile at a slightly faster pace than the first two. If you can't run 3 miles, then run/walk the total distance. After the run, get in the pool and do the following 600-yard workout:
- 100 straight swim, :30 rest
- 6x50 hard, :30 rest
- 100 kick with a kick board and fins if you need them, :30 rest
- 100 straight swim cool-down, swimming as easily as you possibly can

NOTES: _____

If you feel yourself getting intimidated about any parts of the race or course, remember to master your mind, don't let your mind master you. Stay in the moment, relax and remind yourself, "I'm all right, I'm all right."
   —Mark H. Wilson, Race Director of HITS
      Triathlon Series

Week 3

DAY
15
Mon

REST
Fifteen days in, you probably understand why we have these rest days, right?

DAY
16
Tue

BIKE 75-Minute Bike Ride
Go outside and ride, and do the last 15 minutes a little harder than the first 60. If you're indoors, increase the bike resistance for the last 15 minutes to get a similar workout.

DAY
17
Wed

RUN 2-Mile Interval Run
Use the first mile for a warm-up, and then over the next mile focus on running hard 3 intervals of 1 minute each (this would be referred to as 3x1 minute). Work on going from a fast-run interval to slowing back to a jog without walking. If you must walk, then walk to catch your breath and then progress back to a jog and finish the entire 2 miles.

DAY
18
Thu

SWIM 600-Yard Swim
Total workout is 600 yards as follows:
- 50 kick, :30 rest
- 100 swim, :30 rest
- 200 swim/kick (swim down, grab your kick board, kick 2 lengths, drop the board, swim 2 lengths; repeat for 8 lengths total), :30 rest
- 3x50 at a hard intensity, :30 rest
- 100 straight swim as easily as you possibly can go

NOTES: _____

DAY
19
Fri

CROSS-TRAIN   Cross-Training Workout B (page 93)

DAY
20
Sat

BIKE/RUN BRICK   60-Minute Bike Ride; 2-Mile Run
60-minute hard spin class or hilly bike ride, followed by a 2-mile run. Go straight from cycling to running as quickly as possible to begin to get an idea of how it will feel on race day to go from biking to running during T2. This 2-mile run will be a "pickup run," where you increase your pace slightly throughout the entire 2 miles. By the last .25 mile you should be at the pace you hope to run on race day. This is called "race pace." Creative, huh?

DAY
21
Sun

RUN/SWIM BRICK   3-Mile Run; 500-Meter Swim
Try to run the distance at a moderate pace; if you can't run 3 miles yet, then run/walk. Then hop in the pool and do 500 yards (20 lengths) with your choice of drills, duration and rest. However, you want to get it done: Do at least 20 lengths swimming, kicking with fins before you get out of that pool!

NOTES: _____

_____

_____

_____

_____

_____

_____

_____

_____

_____

FROM A TADPOLE TO A SHARK

When I started triathlon, I had never swum, and initially I really wasn't very good at all. Some well-meaning yet misinformed people told me that I would never get good enough to compete at the pro level. Naysayers seemed to come out of the woodwork telling me not to waste my time, and I'm glad I didn't listen. Now that I've been a professional triathlete for over a decade, I've met many people who were in the same situation as me with no swimming background who learned to swim at a very high level. Don't let anyone tell you that it's impossible to improve; through hard work and determination you'll prove them wrong.
        —Lewis

Week 4

DAY
22
Mon

REST

DAY
23
Tue

BIKE   60-Minute Bike Ride

Do 3x3 minutes at your goal race pace for your upcoming tri that's less than a month away! Don't worry, you're doing great and we'll have you ready in time. Rest and pedal easily in between each repeat. Total ride time is 1 hour.

DAY
24
Wed

RUN   2-Mile Interval Run

Do 4x90 seconds at a faster pace: Go from jogging to a faster pace for 90 seconds, and then back to jogging until you recover and can go fast again. Do 4 of these on your 2-mile run.

DAY
25
Thu

SWIM   700-Yard Swim

Total workout is 700 yards as follows:
- 300 (12 lengths) straight swim/kick (wear fins if you need to), :30 rest
- 4x50 hard swimming, :30 rest
- 100 straight swim without stopping, :30 rest
- 50 easy kick, 50 easy swim to cool down

NOTES:

DAY 26 Fri	**CROSS-TRAIN** Cross-Training Program C (page 94)
DAY 27 Sat	**BIKE/RUN BRICK** 75-Minute Bike Ride; 1.5-Mile Run Do the last 15 minutes of the ride at a very hard pace. Followed that up with a 1.5-mile run at a 90% effort of what you think you could do if you went all out. This workout should be very challenging! Make sure you have 1–2 water bottles on the bike and bring 1 along on the run. This workout is to introduce you to threshold training, finding a high intensity that you can maintain for 60–90 minutes.
DAY 28 Sun	**RUN** 4 miles Yesterday was tough, so today shouldn't be. Run/walk if you need to; focus on jogging easily for 4 miles.

NOTES: _____

_____

_____

_____

_____

_____

_____

_____

Warning: Triathlons are extremely addictive, hence the impulse spending on wetsuits, bikes, running shoes, aero bars, aero helmets, speed suits, power meters, GPS heart-rate monitors and many other "gotta have" items.
—Nick Clark, Clark Endurance

Week 5

DAY 29 Mon

REST

DAY 30 Tue

BIKE/RUN BRICK   60-Minute Bike Ride; 1-Mile Run

During the run, do 3x4 minutes at goal race pace. Do easy spinning in between each interval for :30. Follow immediately with an easy run. This will continue to reinforce what it's like to run with wobbly legs off the bike and help you get comfortable feeling like you're running with someone else's legs stitched onto your torso.

DAY 31 Wed

RUN   3-Mile Interval Run

Do 5x60 seconds at a faster pace. Make it continuous running—try not to take any walking breaks, even immediately after the hard efforts. You're working on pacing, and changing speeds while you're running will help you to be able to find your ideal pace even when fatigued.

DAY 32 Thu

SWIM   800-Yard Swim

Total workout is 800 yards as follows:
- 100 easy swim, :30 rest
- 4x75 race pace, :30 rest
- 4x50 above race pace, :30 rest
- 4x25 all-out sprint, :30 rest
- 100 easy swim to cool down

NOTES: _____
_____
_____
_____
_____
_____
_____
_____
_____
_____
_____
_____
_____
_____

DAY **33** Fri	**CROSS-TRAIN** Cross-Training Program A (see page 92)	
DAY **34** Sat	**BIKE/RUN BRICK** 75-Minute Bike Ride; 2-Mile Run During the ride, do 3x5 minutes at goal race pace. For the run, do the first mile easy and the second mile at goal race pace. Don't forget to eat and drink during and after this workout!	
DAY **35** Sun	**RUN** 5-Mile Run No intervals, no pickups, just run as slowly as you need to and get in the miles. Today isn't about speed, it's about getting in shape and just covering the distance.	

NOTES: _____

_____

_____

_____

_____

_____

_____

_____

During a triathlon, if something is working well, keep doing it. If something is wrong, fix it. Above all else, keep moving forward!

Week 6

DAY 36
Mon

REST

Now is a great time to assess how you're feeling about your preparedness; are you ready? If so, then that's awesome, if not—don't stress about it too much. If you've successfully completed even half of the workouts over the previous five weeks you should be A-OK; you'll have done more training than I did for my first triathlon!

DAY 37
Tue

RIDE/RUN BRICK 70-Minute Bike Ride; 2-Mile Run

During the ride, do 3x5 minutes at goal race pace. For the run, do the first .25 mile hard, then jog easily until the last .25 mile, then run that segment hard again.

DAY 38
Wed

RUN 3-Mile Track Workout

880 yards (2 laps), easy, :90 rest
4x880 at above goal race pace, :90 resting; try not to sit down during the rest, just stand. Run all 4 at an uncomfortably fast pace, but try to run each one faster, not slower. This is called a "descending" pace set.
880 yards easy cool-down.

DAY 39
Thu

SWIM 1000-Yard Swim

Total workout is 1000 yards as follows:
- 150 easy straight swim, :30 rest
- 100 easy kick, :30 rest
- 4x100 at race pace, :30 rest
- 4x50 at above race pace, :30 rest
- 50 all-out sprint, :30 rest
- 100 very easy cool-down

NOTES: _____

DAY 40 Fri

CROSS-TRAIN Cross-Training Program B (see page 93)

DAY 41 Sat

BIKE/RUN BRICK 80-Minute Bike Ride; 3-Mile Run
Do the last 20 minutes of your ride at a hard pace, slightly below race pace/effort. For the run, the first 2 miles are easy, then run the final mile at your goal race pace for next weekend.

DAY 42 Sun

RUN 3-Mile Run
This should be an easy run. If you feel good, run the second 1.5 miles up near your goal race pace, but certainly not over it. After your run, refuel and re-hydrate. Check out the event's website and make sure you know everything, from the exact driving directions to all the specific instructions you'll need for race day. Check to see if there's an early packet pickup or bike drop-off and plan accordingly.

NOTES: _____

_____

_____

_____

_____

_____

_____

_____

_____

This sport called triathlon becomes a part of you. You start to plan your entire year around sprint, international, half iron- or full iron-distance races. Your vacations become racing, and you start to realize that this could become a lifelong adventure.
—Nick Clark, Clark Endurance

Week 7

DAY
43
Mon

REST

Less than one week until race day. This is the perfect time to go over all of your gear, use the "Triathlon Race Day Checklist" on page 35 or at www.7weekstofitness.com, and make sure you have everything you need and it's all in working order. You've done some fantastic work to get this far by building your body and mind in order to have the necessary strength, skill and confidence on race day.

DAY
44
Tue

BIKE/RUN BRICK 45-Minute Bike Ride; 2-Mile Run

During the ride, do the last 5 minutes at race pace. For the run, do the last .25 mile at race pace. During this workout really visualize yourself racing—focus on that! Get good carbs/protein after this workout right away; recovery is so important now that you're five days away from your race.

DAY
45
Wed

RUN 2-Mile Taper

This is a shorter run workout because you're now "tapering" for the race. During the 2 miles, do 5x:30 pickups. For the pickups, you run a little over race pace, then go back into a jog. You should finish this workout feeling great, like you want to do more—but don't.

DAY
46
Thu

SWIM 600-Yard Taper

Total workout is 600 yards as follows:
- 100 easy swim, :30 rest
- 100 easy kick, :30 rest
- 3x100 at just below or at goal race pace, :30 rest
- 50 fast, slightly above race pace, :30 rest
- 50 easy cool-down

NOTES: _____
_____
_____
_____
_____
_____
_____
_____
_____
_____
_____
_____
_____
_____
_____

DAY
47
Fri

REST

Take it easy during the day and make sure you get a really good night's sleep; two nights before a race it's important to get quality REM sleep for at least 8 hours, as you may not sleep well the night before the race.

DAY
48
Sat

"RACE-PREP" BRICK   20-Minute Bike Ride; 10-Minute Jog

Be sure to do this workout in the morning. The bike ride should be an easy pace with the bicycle "race ready." Do two or three 30-second pickups, going from slow speed up to race pace, and be sure to go through the gears and check the brakes. Everything should feel perfect! Off the bike, do the jog in the race shoes you plan to wear tomorrow.

Double-check that all your race gear is packed and ready to go, then get some good calories in and rest up for the big day tomorrow. Today you may have to attend the race expo for packet pickup and/or to drop your bike off at transition based on the event. Some athletes like to nap in the afternoon before a race because they'll probably be too excited to sleep that night.

DAY
49
Sun

RACE DAY!

Arrive early and plan time for issues because they *always* seem to arise. Remember that today's event is all about having fun and that there's no such thing as a perfect race—do *your personal best*.

NOTES: _____

_____

_____

_____

_____

_____

_____

_____

_____

_____

_____

After Your First Race

Congratulations on completing your first race—now you're a triathlete! Make sure to share your race experiences, tips, tricks, highs and lows with everyone on facebook.com/7weekstoatriathlon. Yes, it's OK to wear your finisher's medal for the rest of the day and at dinner that night. Just remember to change out of your bike shorts; most restaurants frown on such attire.

Take two days completely off from training, then slowly work back into a routine of running two to three times a week, swimming twice a week and maybe a bike ride on the weekends—all at an easy, recreational pace. Let your body fully recover from the race and all the quality training you've put in over the last seven weeks and the rigors of race day.

Now that you're in "race shape," you won't need to pick a race that's 50 or more days away to train for! Simply cut down this program to your desired next race date by trimming days or weeks off the beginning, making sure you keep the taper in place. Continue to use this program for the remainder of your first season and at the beginning of the next few seasons to shake off the rust and get into race shape quickly. Each time you use the program, feel free to bump up the intensity and add more repeats as necessary. For many triathletes who want to focus on shorter distances, this may be the only program

they ever need. When you're ready to move up to longer distances or push yourself to get significantly faster, stronger and more competitive, the Advanced program is waiting for you on the very next page!

Advanced Program

The following program designed for the experienced triathlete looking to become competitive in any distance triathlon, whether it be a blazing-fast PR in a sprint to your first or fastest ultra distance race. This periodized, pro-caliber training plan focuses on middle- and long-course event distances with some single-sport focus weeks. To hit the target for ultra distance training, you can modify this plan by increasing distances by about 20 percent. If you're looking to develop speed and strength to dominate your age group in sprint distances, add some more intensity to every workout and decrease overall workout distances by 10 percent.

This is a demanding program in multiple ways: the workout itself, the time commitment, the focus on equipment and nutrition, as well as the toll all this can take on personal relationships. If you don't have the time to fully commit to this program, you can use the workouts as a guideline and space them farther apart to allow more time for family, work and other obligations. If you do have the time and drive to commit to this program, it can propel you from the middle of the pack to age-group podium faster than you ever thought possible!

Pro Tip #15 is "Join a masters swim class," and that is highly recommended before beginning the Advanced program. The multitude of drills, varying intensity, motivation that you'll get from the other swimmers and all the tips you'll pick up make it worth every penny and a great use of your time. If you choose not to join a masters swim class or one isn't available in your area, log on to www.7weekstofitness.com and view some of the swim drills you can incorporate into your own swim training to use in place of "masters swim" in the program.

Reading the Advanced Charts

"Race pace" refers to your goal pace for racing long course triathlons: a 1.2-mile swim, a 56-mile bike and a 13.1-mile swim.

For repeats and duration like " 0x00," the first number is how many times you'll repeat the drill, and the second

is the duration (distance or time). For example, "8x1 length" means you'll swim 1 length of the pool and repeat 8 times with the desired rest between sets. "3x3 minutes" or "3x3:00" should be read as 3 repeats of that drill for 3 minute durations each time.

When there's no specified amount of rest, the goal is to catch your breath and mentally prepare for the next set; :30 to 1:00 is average. You're training, not dilly-dallying.

"Split brick" refers to workouts in either two or all three triathlon disciplines in one day, though not specifically performed immediately after each other. These are often called 2-a-days or 3-a-days as well.

A "straight" swim means no stopping through the entire distance.

This 7-week program is for experienced triathletes who have competed in multiple events and are looking to push themselves to get faster, stronger and more competitive. A pro-caliber program that was created by a successful professional triathlete with 10 years of experience, this is not intended for beginners and requires a significant amount of time dedicated to physical and mental preparedness.

Week 1

DAY 1 Mon
MASTERS SWIM   3000–4000 Yards

DAY 2 Tue
BIKE/RUN BRICK   90-Minute Bike Ride; 2-Mile Run
Do 15 minutes of the ride near race pace. For the run, do the first mile easy, the second at goal race pace.

DAY 3 Wed
RUN/SWIM SPLIT BRICK
MORNING: Track workout—1-mile warm-up, 4x800 hard with :90 rest between each, 1-mile cool-down.
LUNCH: Masters swim, 3000 yards total

DAY 4 Thu
BIKE AND CROSS-TRAIN   90-Minute Hill Ride; Cross-Training Program A (page 92)
In the morning, try to climb at Olympic-distance goal pace for 20–30 minutes of the bike ride. Cross-train later in the day.

DAY 5 Fri
REST

DAY 6 Sat
BIKE/SWIM SPLIT BRICK
MORNING: 3-hour bike ride, group ride if you like; take on-bike nutrition and keep intensity low to moderate.
AFTERNOON/EVENING: Go for an easy 1500-yard straight swim.

DAY 7 Sun
RUN   9-Mile Run
This is your long run, so take it at an easy pace (about 1:00–1:30 slower than race pace); focus on your running form and breathing.

NOTES:

Week 2

DAY 8 Mon

MASTERS SWIM 3000–4000 Yards

DAY 9 Tue

BIKE/RUN BRICK 100-Minute Bike Ride; 3-Mile Run
Spend 20 minutes of the ride in the aero bars at race pace. For the run, increase pace each mile, with the third mile about :30 faster than race pace.

DAY 10 Wed

RUN/SWIM SPLIT BRICK
MORNING: Track workout—1.5-mile warm-up, 4x1 mile :30 faster than race pace with :90 rest between each; 1 mile easy cool-down.
LUNCH: Masters swim—3000-4000 yards

DAY 11 Thu

BIKE, CROSS-TRAIN 100-Minute Hill Ride; Cross-Training Program B (page 93)
In the morning, ride the hills at or faster than race pace. This should be a hard effort on the bike, more like a race than a ride. Make sure to hydrate during the ride and refuel immediately afterward. Later in the day, perform your cross-training workout with focus on good form for each movement and less on overall intensity. Your morning ride should be the high-octane portion of today's workout, and you should have very little left in your tank.

NOTES: _____
_____
_____
_____
_____
_____
_____
_____
_____
_____
_____
_____
_____

DAY 12 Fri	REST
DAY 13 Sat	**SWIM/BIKE SPLIT BRICK** MORNING: Ride 3.5 hours with at least 1 hour in the aero bars at race pace. AFTERNOON/EVENING: Go for an easy 2000-yard straight swim; focus on stroke efficiency, maximizing distance covered per stroke.
DAY 14 Sun	**RUN** 11-Mile Run Do this long run at an easy pace.

NOTES: _____

_____

_____

_____

_____

_____

_____

_____

Triathlon will change your outlook on life, your career, your marriage, your goals, your friends and many other things you thought you had figured out. It's not just crossing a finish line or going home with a boring medal. It's the countless hours that got you to that point—a moment in time that you'll never forget, a moment that you'll discuss with your family and friends for hours if not days after the event. These discussions will most likely be about how you could've done better: At what point could you have swum faster, biked harder or ran more efficiently? This is what'll go through your head every day until you get the opportunity to suffer again.

—Nick Clark, Clark Endurance

Week 3: Swim Focus Week

DAY
15
Mon

MASTERS SWIM 4000 Yards

DAY
16
Tue

BIKE/RUN/SWIM SPLIT BRICK
MORNING: Bike 75 minutes at a moderate pace immediately followed by a 3-mile moderate run. For both, your effort level should be less than actual race effort; your run should be about :30 slower than race pace. You'll finish the brick tired, but not totally gassed.
AFTERNOON/EVENING: Masters swim, 4000 yards.

DAY
17
Wed

RUN/SWIM SPLIT BRICK
MORNING: Track workout—1-mile warm-up, 8x400s fast with :90 seconds rest, 1-mile cool-down.
AFTERNOON/EVENING: Masters swim, 3000 yards.

DAY
18
Thu

SWIM/BIKE SPLIT BRICK
MORNING: Masters swim (3000–4000 yards) plus an easy 45-minute bike ride or spin class.
AFTERNOON/EVENING: Masters swim, 4000 yards.

NOTES: _____
_____
_____
_____
_____
_____
_____
_____
_____
_____
_____
_____
_____

DAY 19 Fri	REST
DAY 20 Sat	**BIKE/SWIM SPLIT BRICK** MORNING: Long ride of 3.5 hours at moderate intensity; group ride possible here. AFTERNOON/EVENING: 2500-yard swim at moderate intensity, slightly slower than race pace.
DAY 21 Sun	**RUN/SWIM BRICK** 12-Mile Run; 2000-Yard Swim For this long run, go 1:00–1:30 slower than race pace. The swim should be at a moderate pace.

NOTES: _____

_____

_____

_____

_____

_____

_____

_____

I was training with a top triathlon coach a few years ago during the off-season. I told him I was just off the main pack in most of the long and ultra-distance triathlons, and that I was hoping to close this gap somehow. He gave me 10 tips for faster swimming. It turns out I was incorporating six or seven of them into my everyday training, but three or four of them I had yet to apply, or didn't do regularly. For the next three months I made sure I went 10 for 10, and the following year I posted my best swim splits yet, including a 24:28 for 1.2 miles at the Wildflower Triathlon.
    —Lewis

Week 4: Bike Focus Week

DAY 22
Mon

SWIM/BIKE BRICK   3000–4000-Yard Masters Swim;
60-Minute Bike Ride
The ride should be at a very easy recovery pace. This ride is to loosen up your legs and hips to prepare for the rigors of the bike focus week.

DAY 23
Tue

BIKE/RUN BRICK   2-Hour Bike Ride; 2-Mile Run
During the ride, do 3x10 minutes faster than race pace while on the aero bars. The run should be at a moderate effort, about 1:00 slower than race pace.

DAY 24
Wed

RIDE/SWIM SPLIT BRICK   2.5-Hour Bike Ride;
3000- to 4000-Yard Masters Swim OR 2200-Yard Straight Swim
During the ride, do 2x20:00 at race pace on the aero bars. Finish the ride with one-legged-drills: Pedal 60 revolutions with one leg on the pedal, the other "clipped" out off to the side, then do the other leg. Repeat 3 times with each leg. Try to keep even-pressure throughout the whole rotation with no jumps in chain tension; the bike should just roll smoothly. Pedal all 360 degrees!
    If you're doing the straight swim, do 8x25 yards slightly faster than race pace.

DAY 25
Thu

BIKE, CROSS-TRAIN   2.5-Hour Hill Ride;
Cross-Training Program C (page 94)
This ride is going to rely heavily on the topography, and you may need to loop around a bit to make sure you get the hill work done. Do 4x5:00 in the saddle, just below race pace intensity at around 40–50 cadence (or crank revolutions per minute). These are called "strength endurance intervals" or "hill repeats." But you can call them by their other name, the Devil. Follow up later in the day with the cross-training workout. Luckily, you have a rest day tomorrow.

NOTES: _____

_____

_____

_____

_____

_____

_____

_____

_____

_____

_____

_____

_____

DAY
26
Fri

REST

DAY
27
Sat

BIKE/SWIM SPLIT BRICK

MORNING: 4-hour bike ride on your own or with a group. Do 90 minutes at or just below race pace and get in the aero bars as often as you can while being as safe as possible; going aero can be a little intimidating in a fast paceline or around a group, but it's a skill you'll need to learn to be an elite triathlete.
AFTERNOON/EVENING: Hit the pool for an easy 1500-yard straight recovery swim.

DAY
28
Sun

RUN/BIKE SPLIT BRICK   13-Mile Run; 1-Hour Bike Ride

For this long run, go very easy, 1:30–2:00 per mile slower than race pace. After refueling, later in the day take the bike out for an easy recovery ride at an easy pace with a very low heart rate. Just spin an easy gear here to shake out your legs after a tough week on the bike!

NOTES: _____

_____

_____

_____

_____

_____

_____

_____

_____

Week 5: Run Focus Week

DAY
29
Mon

MASTERS SWIM 3000–4000 Yards
Keep the intensity low, just get in the distance. This may require you to join a slower group than you normally would!

DAY
30
Tue

BIKE/RUN BRICK 60-Minute Bike Ride; 45-Minute Run
The ride should be an easy pace. Follow it up with the run at a moderate pace, :15–:30 per mile slower than race pace.

DAY
31
Wed

RUN/SWIM SPLIT BRICK
MORNING: Track Workout—the fabled Yasso 800s! These are the run workouts long heralded for their difficulty and high rate of success in building faster runners. They start with a 2-mile warm-up, then 10x800 yards at or faster than race pace, with 2:00 rest between each, and a 1–2 mile cool-down.

Refuel and rest, and later on go for an easy 2000- to 3000-yard recovery straight swim.

DAY
32
Thu

BIKE/RUN BRICK, CROSS-TRAIN 60-Minute Bike Ride; 60-Minute Run
Start with a 60-minute bike ride, perform the final 15 minutes of the ride at race pace, with the rest easy to moderate. Follow that with a 60-minute run, doing the first 40 minutes at :30 per mile faster than race pace; run the last 20 minutes at race pace. Yes, you should be exhausted after this workout, but each time you push your limits you raise your future performance potential.

After resting and refueling, later that day perform Cross-Training Program A (see page 92) at moderate intensity with a careful focus on warm-up, exercise form and stretching.

NOTES:

DAY 33 Fri	**REST**
DAY 34 Sat	**BIKE/RUN/SWIM SPLIT BRICK** MORNING: 90- to 120-minute bike ride, moderate to low intensity, immediately followed by an easy 2-mile run. AFTERNOON/EVENING: Follow it all up later in the day with an easy 2000-yard swim.
DAY 35 Sun	**RUN** 15 Miles OR 2 Hours, whichever comes first This is your long run, so go easy, bring nutrition, and get in good calories/fluids immediately after for fast recovery!

NOTES: _____
_____
_____
_____
_____
_____
_____
_____

WTC is by far the largest and most recognized brand in triathlon events, and the Ironman name and logo are woven tightly into the fabric of the sport; getting WTC's Ironman "M-Dot" logo tattooed on an Ironman finisher's calf has become a rite of passage for many. That doesn't mean WTC events are the only triathlons to be found—not by a long shot. Thousands of swim, bike and run events are held all over the world each year by individuals, groups, charities and organizations large and small.

Week 6

DAY 36 Mon	**BIKE/SWIM SPLIT BRICK** MORNING: Very easy 45-minute bike ride. This recovery ride should be done at a low heart rate; spin as easy a gear as you can to shake your legs out. AFTERNOON/EVENING: Perform an easy 1500-yard swim at a slow "recovery" pace.
DAY 37 Tue	**BIKE/RUN BRICK** 90-Minute Bike Ride; 4-Mile Run During the ride, do 3x10 minutes at race pace. For the run, do the first mile easy, second mile at race pace and the third mile :30 faster than race pace. Cool down with a 1-mile run about 1:00 slower than race pace.
DAY 38 Wed	**RUN/SWIM SPLIT BRICK** MORNING: Track Workout—1-mile warm-up, 2x800 with 1 minute rest between, 4x400 with 90 seconds rest between, 4x200 with 60 seconds rest between, 1-mile cool-down. AFTERNOON/EVENING: Later in the day hit the pool for a masters swim, 3000–4000 yards total.
DAY 39 Thu	**BIKE, CROSS-TRAIN** 90-Minute Bike Ride; Cross-Training Program B (page 93) The ride should be hilly, at a moderate intensity. Finish this ride wanting to do more—but don't. Later in the day, perform Cross-Training Workout B; focus on warm-up, exercise form and stretching.

NOTES: _____

_____

_____

_____

_____

_____

_____

_____

_____

_____

_____

		NOTES: _____
DAY **40** Fri	REST	

DAY **41** Sat — **BIKE/SWIM SPLIT BRICK**
MORNING: 2-hour bike ride with 2x10 minutes at race pace on the aero bars.
AFTERNOON: Swim an easy 1000 yards in the pool.

DAY **42** Sun — **RUN**   8- to 9-Mile Run
This run should be at an easy to moderate pace about 1:00 slower than race pace. You should finish feeling like you could run more, but don't exceed this distance.

Swim 2.4 miles! Bike 112 miles! Run 26.2 miles! Brag for the rest of your life.™
—Commander John Collins, organizer of the first Ironman event

Week 7: Taper Week

DAY
43
Mon

REST

DAY
44
Tue

BIKE/RUN BRICK   60-Minute Bike Ride; 10-Minute Run
Do the ride easy. During the run, do 4x30 second pickups—lift the pace to very brisk, but only for 30 seconds, then back to a jog.

DAY
45
Wed

RUN   Track Workout
Do a 1-mile warm-up, 2x800, 2x400, 2x200, all with 60 seconds rest, at about 80-percent effort level. Leave something in the tank! Finish with a 1-mile cool-down.

DAY
46
Thu

BIKE/SWIM BRICK   60-Minute Bike Ride; 1500- to 2000-Yard Swim
Use the bike you're racing this weekend for an easy ride and check the entire bike to make sure it's race ready! Follow that with an easy swim, and be sure to do 4x100-yard repeats at race pace.

NOTES: _____

_____

_____

_____

_____

_____

_____

_____

_____

_____

		NOTES: _____
DAY 47 Fri	**REST** Hydrate, eat and stretch lightly throughout the day. Make sure to get at least 8 hours of quality REM sleep tonight; you may not sleep very well the night before the race.	_____
DAY 48 Sat	**BIKE/RUN/SWIM SPLIT BRICK** MORNING: 30-minute easy bike ride on race-ready bike. Follow with a 10-minute easy run while adding in 2–3 :30 pick-ups at race pace. After a short rest, hop in the pool for a 300- to 500-yard easy swim with 4x25 at race intensity; the rest just long, easy strokes. Get this all done in the morning and then double-check all your gear and head down to your race venue/expo and check your bike and bags in if you need to. Once you get home, put your feet up and relax—take an afternoon nap if you can!	
DAY 49 Sun	**RACE!**	

Congratulations on your big race! Here's hoping that all your hard work, training and preparation paid off with a new personal best and the desire to continue pushing your goals higher. You can modify the time frame and intensity of the Advanced Program to fit your race schedule by trimming weeks off the front of the program, keeping the race prep and taper intact. As you progress, push the intensity of the program by lowering your race pace to the best of your ability. If you're setting the bar really high, check out "So You're Thinking about Going Pro" on page 51; you might just have what it takes to join the ranks of the elite professional multisport athletes!

For additional pro-caliber swim workouts created by masters swim coach Frank Sole, visit www.7weeksoffitness.com

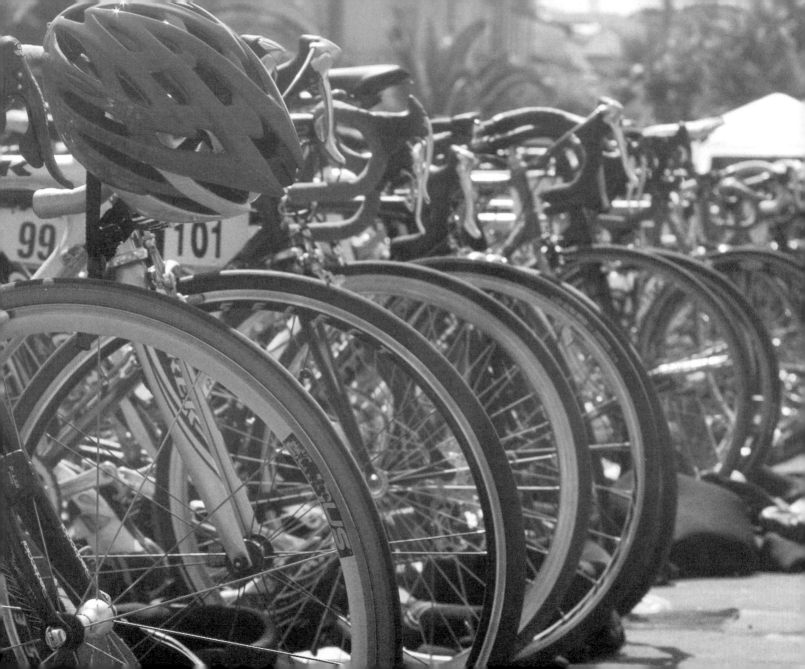

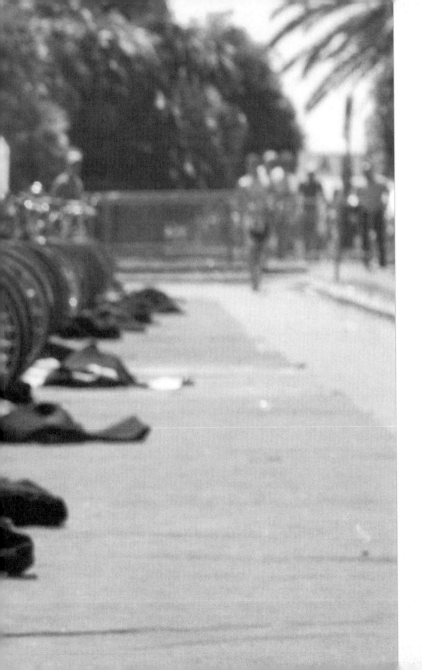

PART 3:
BEYOND THE
PROGRAM

Cross-Training for Triathlon Success

The sport of triathlon itself is fantastic cross-training for nearly any other sport or activity; by combining the disciplines of swimming, biking and running you're performing multiple movements in various planes to target the entire body to build power, speed, endurance and—more importantly—strengthen weaknesses and imbalances that your body has developed from performing one sport.

Functional cross-training exercises in conjunction with the triathlon training programs in this book will take your fitness to a whole new level. By incorporating full-range-of-motion bodyweight exercises along with high-intensity intervals, multi-joint movements and stretches into your training, you can develop a new level of total-body fitness that will translate directly into triathlon success!

This workout plan is designed to complement and not replace the discipline-specific Beginner or Advanced 7 Weeks to a Triathlon training plans when performed in-season and during race preparation. In the off-season, you can ratchet up the intensity by adding exercise reps and sets, and even sprint intervals and long runs, to this cross-training program.

Warming Up and Stretching

Properly warming up the body prior to any activity is very important, as is stretching post-workout. Please note that warming up and stretching are two completely different things: A warm-up routine should be done before stretching so that your muscles are more pliable and able to be stretched efficiently. You should not "warm up" by stretching; you simply don't want to push, pull or stretch cold muscles.

It's crucial to raise your body temperature prior to beginning a workout. In order to prevent injury, such as a muscle strain, you want to loosen up your muscles and joints before you begin the actual exercise movement. A good warm-up before your workout should slowly raise your core body temperature, heart rate and breathing. Before jumping into the workout, you must increase blood flow to all working areas of the body. This augmented blood flow will transport more oxygen and nutrients to the muscles being worked. The warm-up will also increase the range of motion of your joints.

A warm-up should consist of light physical activity (such as walking, jogging in place, stationary biking, jumping jacks, etc.) and only take between 5–10 minutes to complete. Your individual fitness level and the activity determine how hard and how long you should go but, generally speaking, the average person should build up to a light sweat during warm-up. You want to prepare your body for activity, not fatigue it.

Stretching should generally be done after a workout. It'll help you reduce soreness from the workout, increase range of motion and flexibility within a joint or muscle, and prepare your body for any future workouts. Stretching immediately post- exercise while your muscles are still warm allows your muscles to return to their full range of motion (which gives you more flexibility gains) and reduces the chance of injury or fatigue in the hours or days after an intense workout. It's important to remember that even when you're warm and loose, you should never "bounce" during stretching. Keep your movements slow and controlled.

Note: Start with a 5-minute warm-up (see pages 119–23). Perform 4 rounds total for each program. Finish with a 5-minute cool-down and 5 minutes of stretching (see pages 124–28).

Cross-Training Program A

Beginner

Set 1	10 Sit-Ups (page 96)	12 Hip Raises (page 102)	12 Mountain Climbers (page 106)
		Rest :30	
Set 2	8 Push-Ups (page 108)	8 Overhead Presses with Band *do reps with one hand, then switch sides* (page 112)	:30 Wall Sit (page 116)
		Rest :30	
Set 3	8 Band Forward Presses *do reps with one hand, then switch sides* (page 114)	10 Stability Ball Reverse Rollers (page 109)	15 Stability Ball Crunches (page 100)
		Rest 2:00	

Advanced

Set 1	25 Sit-Ups (page 96)	28 Hip Raises (page 102)	30 Mountain Climbers (page 106)
		Rest :30	
Set 2	18 Push-Ups (page 108)	14 Overhead Presses with Band *do reps with one hand, then switch sides* (page 112)	1:00 Wall Sit (page 116)
		Rest :30	
Set 3	16 Band Forward Presses *do reps with one hand, then switch sides* (page 114)	15 Stability Ball Reverse Rollers (page 109)	25 Stability Ball Crunches (page 100)
		Rest 2:00	

Note: Start with a 5-minute warm-up (see pages 119–23). Perform 4 rounds total for each program. Finish with a 5-minute cool-down and 5 minutes of stretching (see pages 124–28).

Cross-Training Program B

Beginner

Set 1	12 Reverse Crunches (page 97)	10 Bird Dogs (page 104)	10 Supermans (page 105)
		Rest :30	
Set 2	3–5 Pull-Ups (page 111)	10 Band Squat and Rows (page 115)	12 Forward Lunges (page 118)
		Rest :30	
Set 3	15 Stability Ball Crunches (page 100)	8 Suspended Hip Bridges (page 103)	10 Stability Ball Extensions (page 110)
		Rest 2:00	

Advanced

Set 1	22 Reverse Crunches (page 97)	20 Bird Dogs (page 104)	22 Supermans (page 105)
		Rest :30	
Set 2	6–10 Pull-Ups (page 111)	22 Band Squat and Rows (page 115)	20 Forward Lunges (page 118)
		Rest :30	
Set 3	25 Stability Ball Crunches (page 100)	16 Suspended Hip Bridges (page 103)	15 Stability Ball Extensions (page 110)
		Rest 2:00	

Note: Start with a 5-minute warm-up (see pages 119–23). Perform 4 rounds total for each program. Finish with a 5-minute cool-down and 5 minutes of stretching (see pages 124–28).

Cross-Training Program C

Beginner

Set 1	12 Bicycle Crunches (page 98)	10 Stability Ball Hip Raises (page 101)	12 Mountain Climbers (page 106)
		Rest :30	
Set 2	10 Band Pull-Downs (page 113)	10 Push-Ups (page 108)	10 Squats (page 117)
		Rest :30	
Set 3	8 Band Forward Presses *do reps with one hand, then switch sides* (page 114)	8 Overhead Presses with Band *do reps with one hand, then switch sides* (page 112)	10 Band Squat and Rows (page 115)
		Rest 2:00	

Advanced

Set 1	22 Bicycle Crunches (page 98)	25 Stability Ball Hip Raises (page 101)	30 Mountain Climbers (page 106)
		Rest :30	
Set 2	18 Band Pull-Downs (page 113)	22 Push-Ups (page 108)	25 Squats (page 117)
		Rest :30	
Set 3	16 Band Forward Presses *do reps with one hand, then switch sides* (page 114)	14 Overhead Presses with Band *do reps with one hand, then switch sides* (page 112)	22 Band Squat and Rows (page 115)
		Rest 2:00	

Cross-Training Exercises

The following exercises make up the functional cross-training component of the 7 Weeks to a Triathon programs. Designed specifically to complement the Beginner and Advanced programs, these moves will help you develop the necessary strength, flexibility, agility and stamina to perform your best on race day.

Sit-Ups

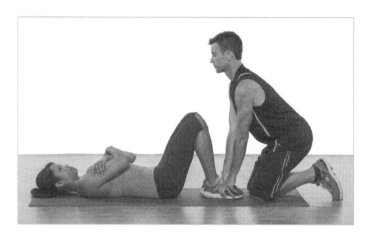

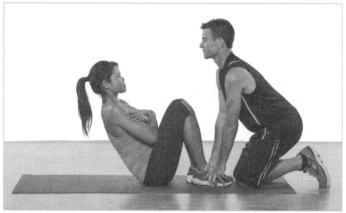

1 On a padded surface, lie face-up with your knees bent to about 90°. Using a partner or fixed object, restrain your feet so they remain flat on the floor during the entire movement. Rest your head, shoulders and back on the floor, and maintain proper curvature of your lower spine, not allowing it to touch the floor. Set your timer for 2 minutes. Cross your arms across your chest with your hands palm-down.

2 Exhale and contract your abdominal muscles to slowly lift your head, arms and upper back off the floor in a controlled manner. Keep your upper back and neck straight and maintain your hand and arm position through the movement. Stop when your back is at about a 45° angle to the floor. Pause briefly and slowly return to starting position.

Reverse Crunch

How do you get all the core-strengthening benefits of a crunch with very limited stress on the lower back? Reverse crunches are the answer! Keep your back straight and lower legs on a level plane throughout this slow and controlled movement.

1 Lie flat on your back with your legs extended along the floor and your arms along your sides, palms down.

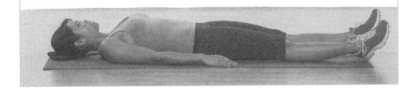

2 Contracting your lower abdominal muscles, lift your feet 4–6 inches off the floor, bend your knees and bring them in toward your chest. Be careful not to put excessive pressure on your lower back by bringing your hips off the floor. Pause when your glutes rise slightly off the mat.

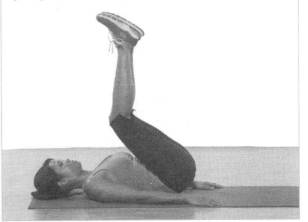

3 Extend your legs and lower them until your feet are 4–6 inches off the floor.

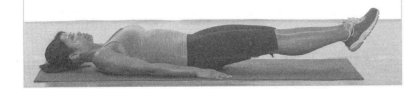

Bicycle Crunch

Rated by the American Council on Exercise as the number-one way to target the rectus abdominis, this move gets your whole body in motion and really works the entire core.

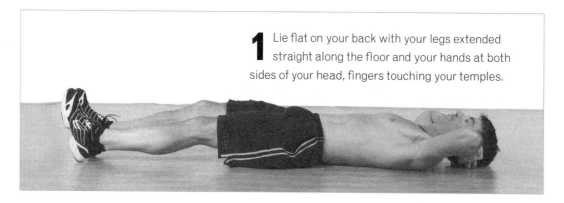

1 Lie flat on your back with your legs extended straight along the floor and your hands at both sides of your head, fingers touching your temples.

2 Raise your feet 6 inches off the floor while simultaneously contracting your rectus abdominis and lifting your upper back and shoulders off the floor. In one movement, bend your left knee and raise your left leg so that the thigh and shin are at 90°; rotate your torso using your oblique muscles so that your right elbow touches the inside of your left knee.

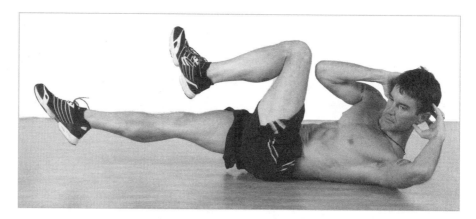

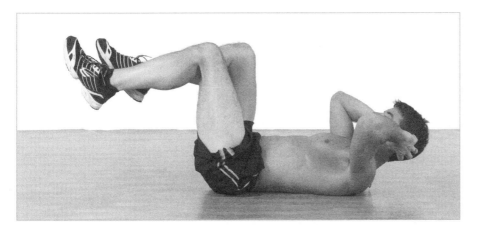

3 Rotate your torso back to center and lower your upper body toward the floor, stopping before your shoulders touch.

4 Extend your left knee and return your foot to 6 inches off the floor and bend your right leg to 90°. Contract your abs, rotate and touch your left elbow to the inside of your right knee. That's 2 reps.

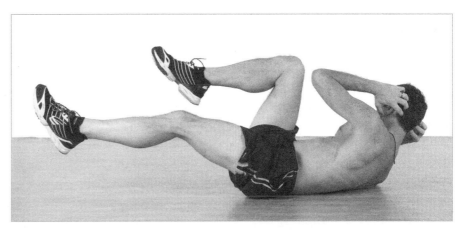

Stability Ball Crunch

The imbalanced platform of the stability ball (shouldn't it be called an instability ball?) helps to activate more of the tiny supporting muscles throughout your core, legs and upper body while it also provides a comfortable base for crunches. The size and shape of the ball also allow you to adjust the difficulty of the crunch and range of motion depending on where you position the ball under your back.

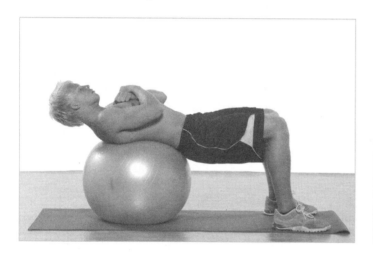 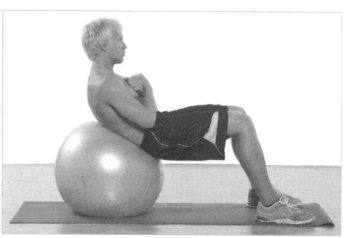

1 Sit on the edge of a stability ball, then lean back and allow the ball to roll forward until it's positioned under your lower back; you'll need to adjust your feet accordingly. Choose your hand position; the farther you place your hands away from your hips, the harder the movement. Start with your arms extended straight with your hands by your hips. If that's too easy, you can cross your arms across your chest or even extend your arms straight over your head. Don't interlock your fingers behind your head; that causes strain on the upper back and neck.

2 Contract your abdominal muscles and lift your shoulder blades off the ball; this is the "up" position. Pause for 1–3 seconds, then slowly return back to starting position.

That's 1 rep.

Stability Ball Hip Raise

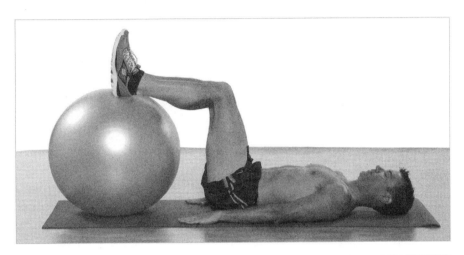

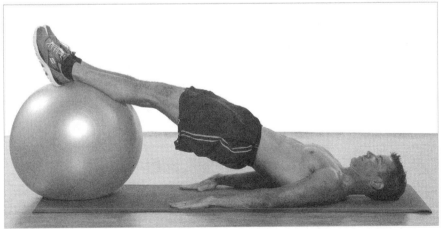

1 Lying on your back, bend your knees and raise your legs high enough to roll a stability ball under your heels. Rest both heels directly on top of the ball 3–6 inches apart. Both knees should be bent 90° and the entire weight of your legs should be resting on the ball. Extend your hands toward your hips and place your arms and palms flat on the floor at your sides.

2 Engage your abdominal muscles to keep your core tight, and exhale while you press your heels into the ball and roll it away from your body. Raise your hips and lower back, forming a straight line from your sternum to your feet while keeping the tops of your shoulder blades flat on the floor. Do not push your hips too high or arch your back. Hold this position for 3–5 seconds, then inhale and slowly roll the ball back toward your butt with your heels and lower yourself back to starting position.

That's 1 rep.

Hip Raise

This exercise is a slow and controlled motion that works the entire core—back, hips and abs—and provides a great way to work those muscles without any impact.

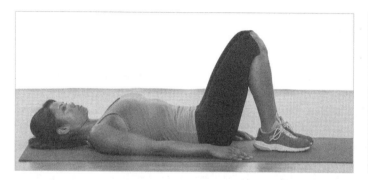

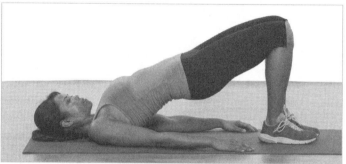

1 Lie on your back with your knees bent and feet flat on the floor, as close to your butt as possible. Extend your hands toward your hips and place your arms and palms flat on the floor at your sides.

2 Engage your abdominal muscles to keep your core tight, and exhale while you press your feet into the floor and raise your hips and lower back up, forming a straight line from your sternum to your knees. Do not push your hips too high or arch your back. Hold this position for 3–5 seconds, and then inhale and slowly return to starting position.

That's 1 rep.

ADVANCED VARIATION: To work your core and stabilizers even more, when your hips reach the top of the motion and your body is flat from sternum to knees, raise one foot off the floor and extend it in front of you in the same line with your torso. Alternate legs with each repetition.

Suspended Hip Bridge

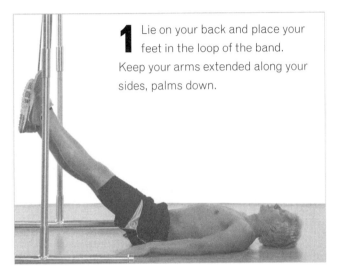

1 Lie on your back and place your feet in the loop of the band. Keep your arms extended along your sides, palms down.

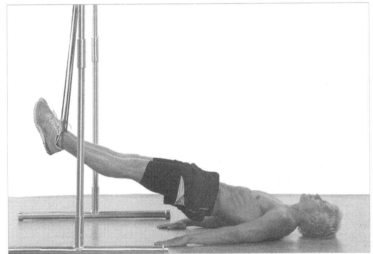

2 Raise your butt off the floor, and then raise your hips and lower back, forming a straight line from your sternum to your feet with the tops of your shoulder blades flat on the floor. Do not push your hips too high or arch your back. Engage your core and squeeze your glutes to keep your back and hips rigid and flat. Hold this position for 3–5 seconds.

In a slow and controlled motion, lower down to starting position. That's 1 rep.

Be careful not to swing or bounce on the exercise band; this should be a very slow and controlled movement with your abs and glutes engaged the entire time.

Bird Dog

The bird dog is an excellent exercise for developing abdominal and hip strength and flexibility, and also for working your lower back by stabilizing your spine throughout the movement.

1 Get on your hands and knees with your legs bent 90°, knees under your hips, toes on the floor and your hands on the floor directly below your shoulders. Keep your head and spine neutral; do not let your head lift or sag. Contract your abdominal muscles to prevent your back from sagging; keep your back flat from shoulders to butt for the entire exercise.

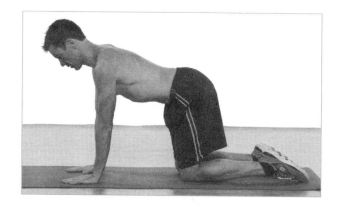

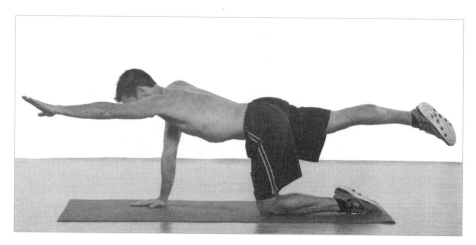

2 In one slow and controlled motion, simultaneously raise your right leg and left arm until they're on the same flat plane as your back. Your leg should be parallel to the ground, not raised above your hip; your arm should extend directly out from your shoulder and your biceps should be level with your ear. Hold this position for 3–5 seconds and then slowly lower your arm and leg back to starting position.

That's 1 rep. Switch sides and repeat.

Superman

Interestingly enough, this exercise is not performed "up, up and away" but actually on your stomach, flat on the ground. However, the Man of Steel would greatly appreciate the importance of this move as it strengthens your lower back and gives some due attention to your erector spinae—you know, those muscles that keep you vertical.

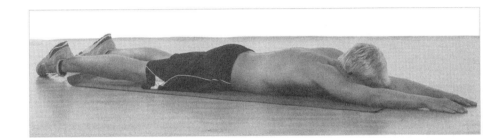

1 Lying face down on your stomach, extend your arms directly out in front of you and your legs behind you. Keep your knees straight as if you were flying.

2 In a slow and controlled manner, contract your erector spinae and reach your arms forward and legs backward toward opposite walls, and allow your arms and feet to raise 3–5 inches off the floor. Your head should maintain a straight position with your spine; do not arch your back. This move is as much of a "stretch" as it is an exercise. Hold for 1–3 seconds.

Lower slowly back to starting position.

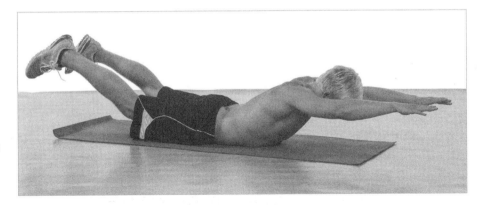

Mountain Climbers

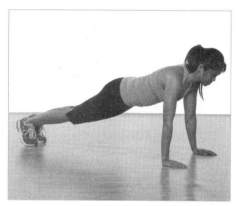
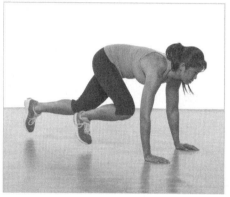
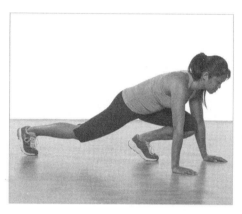

1 Assume the top position of a push-up with your hands directly under your shoulders and toes on the ground. Keep your core engaged and your body in a straight line from head to toe.

2 Lift your right toe slightly off the ground, bring your right knee to your chest and place your right foot on the ground under your body.

3 With a very small hop from both toes, extend your right foot back to starting position and at the same time bring your left knee to your chest and place your left foot on the ground under your body.

Continue switching, making sure to keep your hips low.

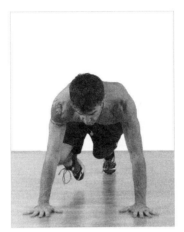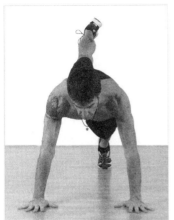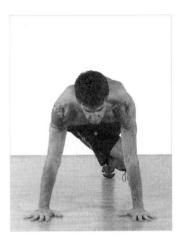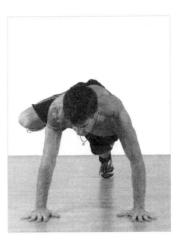

ADVANCED VARIATION: This advanced move really works the core (it's essentially a plank with a lot of leg movement) and strengthens your glutes and hips. Instead of hopping and switching your legs, you'll bring your right knee toward your right shoulder and then extend it straight out behind you (this is the "mule kick," so lift your foot as high as possible while keeping your hips firmly in place; do not rock or raise your butt!). Without touching your foot to the ground, bring your right knee toward your left shoulder before extending it for another mule kick. Lastly, raise your leg laterally (picture a male dog around a fire hydrant) and bring your knee toward your right shoulder, then finish the move with yet another mule kick before returning your right foot back to starting position. Now repeat with your left leg.

Push-Up

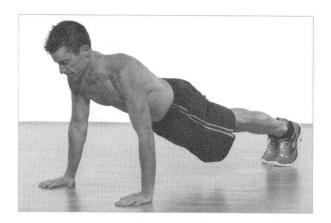

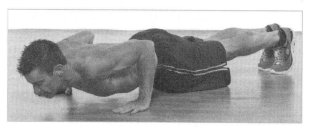

1 Place your hands on the ground approximately shoulder-width apart, making sure your fingers point straight ahead and your arms are straight but your elbows not locked. Step your feet back until your body forms a straight line from head to feet. Your feet should be about 6 inches apart with the weight in the balls of your feet. Engage your core to keep your spine from sagging; don't sink into your shoulders.

2 Inhale as you lower your torso to the ground and focus on keeping your elbows as close to your sides as possible, stopping when your elbows are at a 90° angle or your chest is 1–2 inches from the floor. Pause briefly.

Using your shoulders, chest and triceps, exhale and push your torso back up to starting position.

STAGGERED VARIATION: Staggered push-ups can be done with your hands in pretty much any position as long as you can support yourself. Be aware of any pain in your elbows or shoulders; moving your hands away from your torso increases the load these joints need to bear to lower and raise your body.

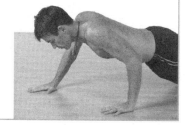

Stability Ball Reverse Roller

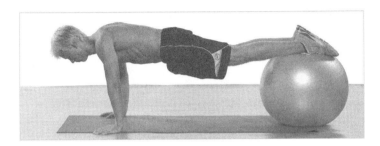

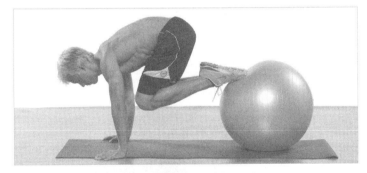

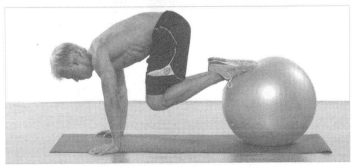

1 Starting on your hands and knees, place the tops of both feet on top of a stability ball. Place your weight in your hands and lift your knees off the mat, balancing your weight on your hands and the stability ball. Walk your hands out until your body forms a straight line from head to feet, engaging your core and glutes to keep your back flat. Your hands should be on the floor just a little bit wider than your shoulders and your neck should be in a neutral position with your head neither raised nor chin pressed to chest.

2 Keeping your back flat and spine straight, exhale and slowly bring your knees in toward your chest and your heels toward your butt. Do not raise your hips or arch your back. Stop when you can't bring your knees any closer toward your chest, and hold that position for 3–5 seconds.

3 In a slow and controlled motion, inhale and extend your legs backward, returning your body to starting position. Be careful not to bounce on the stability ball. This should be a very slow and controlled movement with your abs and glutes engaged the entire time.

That's 1 rep.

Stability Ball Extension

Strengthening the lower back muscles is an extremely important part of core development. In the quest to build six-pack abs, most people focus on the abdominal muscles and fail to properly work the lower back muscles, which often leads to lower back pain. This exercise is one of the simplest ways to build lower back strength and flexibility.

1 Kneeling on the floor, place a stability ball in front of you and lean your upper body forward so your torso rounds over the top of the ball. Roll forward about 2 inches while keeping the ball in contact with your thighs; your hips should now be at about a 100–110° angle. Extend your hands straight out in front of you with your arms alongside your head so your biceps are next to your ears.

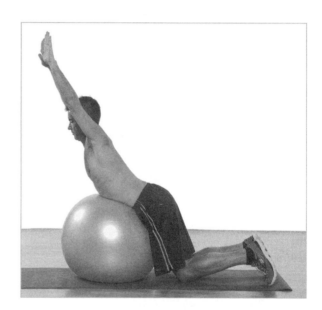

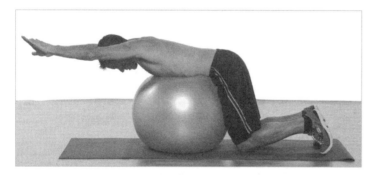

MODIFICATION: For a less-challenging variation, keep your hands on the floor while you position yourself on the ball. When you raise your chest off the ball, extend your arms back toward your hips, alongside your body with your palms facing downward.

2 Once you're positioned on the ball and stable, contract the muscles of your lower back to raise your chest and sternum off the ball and straighten your back. Pause for 1–3 seconds and slowly return to starting position, trying not to bounce off the ball for each motion. That's 1 rep.

Pull-Up

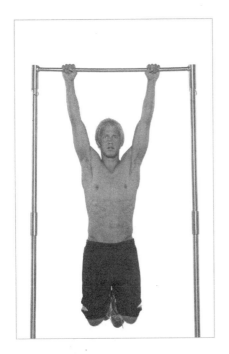

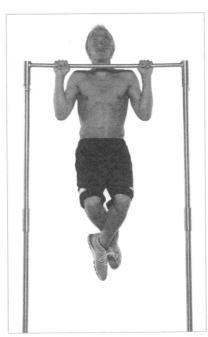

1 Grip the horizontal bar with your palms facing away from you and your arms fully extended. Your hands should be slightly wider (up to 2 inches) than your shoulders. Your feet should not touch the floor during this exercise. Let all of your weight settle in position but don't relax your shoulders—this may cause them to overstretch.

2 Squeeze your shoulder blades together (scapular retraction) to start the initial phase of the pull-up. During this initial movement, pretend that you're squeezing a pencil between your shoulder blades—don't let the pencil drop during any phase of the pull-up. For phase two (upward/concentric phase), look up at the bar, exhale and pull your chin up toward the bar by driving your elbows toward your hips. It's very important to keep your shoulders back and chest up during the entire movement. Pull yourself up in a controlled manner until the bar is just above the top of your chest.

Inhale and lower yourself back to starting position.

Overhead Press with Band

You can control the difficulty of this movement by grasping the band closer to its origin, thereby shortening its length and requiring more force to stretch it to achieve the full range of motion for this exercise.

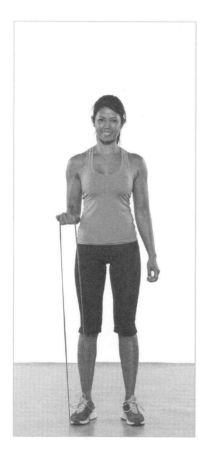

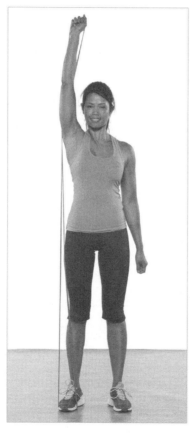

1 Stand up straight with your feet shoulder-width apart and toes pointing forward. Place the lower loop of an exercise band underneath the ball of your right foot and grasp the upper loop of the band with your right hand, palm up, and close your hand firmly around the band. Keeping your elbow tight to your side, bend your elbow and raise your hand up until your forearm is parallel to the floor. The band should be straight but not under much tension. This is your starting position.

2 Perform a biceps curl by keeping your elbow in position and raising your fist toward your right shoulder. As your hand reaches your shoulder, simultaneously rotate your wrist so your palm faces away from your body and press your arm straight up overhead. Finish with your biceps next to your ear and your elbow fully extended but not locked. Slowly reverse the movement and return to starting position.

Repeat for the indicated number of reps with your right arm, then switch the band to your left foot and hand and repeat.

Band Pull-Down

Before starting this exercise, affix the bands securely by looping them around a fixed object overhead like a pull-up bar. If you have only one band, you can perform this movement one side at a time. You can control the tension of the band for this movement by stepping forward or backward.

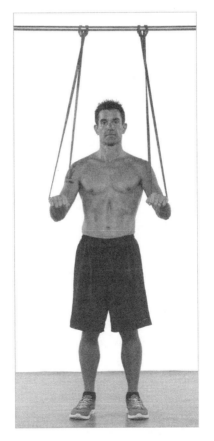 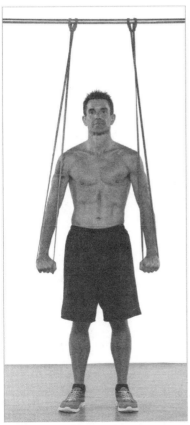

1 Grab the lower loops of the hanging bands with each hand and step backward 2–4 feet from the point at which the bands are attached; the bands should have enough tension to straighten out but not be fully stretched. Facing the bands' attachment points, rotate your hands so your palms face down, and close your grip around the bands. Your feet should be slightly wider than shoulder-width apart and both knees should be bent slightly so you can bend at the waist and lean forward to place your weight on the balls of both feet. This is your starting position.

2 With your elbows straight but not locked, pull the bands in an arc down toward the floor and continue the motion until your arms are behind your body as far as your range of motion or the bands' tension will allow. Engage your core to prevent your body from twisting as you stretch the band in a semicircle. Hold the band in the fully stretched position for 3–5 seconds, then slowly return to starting position.

That's 1 rep; repeat for the indicated number of reps.

Band Forward Press

Before beginning this exercise, affix the band securely to a wall or use a partner to hold it at the same height as your elbow while standing upright. You can control the tension of the band for this movement by stepping forward or backward.

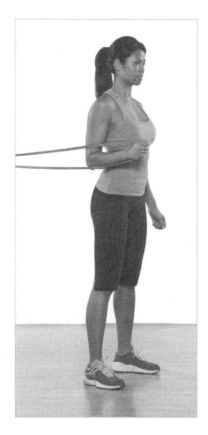

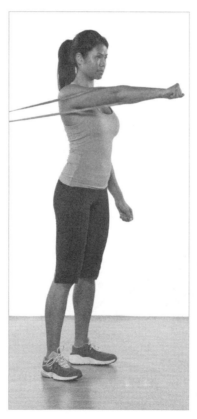

1 Facing away from the band's mount or your partner, grip the open loop of the band with your right hand and walk forward 2–4 feet until the band is straightened but not under much tension. Keeping your knees slightly bent and your left arm extended straight down your body with your palm facing your left thigh, keep your right elbow tight to your body and raise your hand so your right forearm is at a 90° angle relative to your torso. This is your starting position.

2 Engage your core to keep your body from twisting, and extend your arm straight out in front of your body in a controlled "punching" motion, ending when your elbow is fully extended but not locked and your arm is on a level plane with your shoulder. Do not overextend your shoulder; your upper body should remain square in relation to your right arm. Hold this fully stretched position for 3–5 seconds, then slowly return to starting position.

That's 1 rep; repeat for the indicated number of reps before carefully stepping backward to release tension band and swapping hands.

Band Squat and Row

Prior to starting this exercise, attach the band securely to a stable mounting point approximately 30 inches off the ground; optimal height will be level with your chest when you're in the lowest point of a squat with your thighs parallel to the ground. This exercise can also be performed by using a partner to stretch the band at the appropriate height.

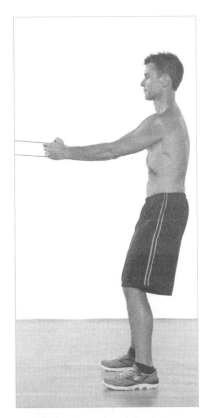

1 Standing erect while facing the mounting point, hold the band in both hands with your arms straight out in front of you at chest height and take 2–3 steps backward to take up any slack in the band. You should look like a water skier holding a tow rope; that's the appropriate starting position for this exercise.

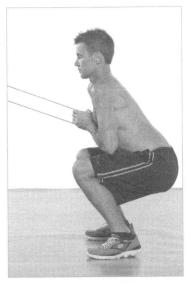

2 With your arms straight out in front of you and both hands grasping the band approximately 8 inches apart with your palms facing the floor, bend your knees and sit back slightly as you lower yourself into a bodyweight squat (page 117). When your thighs are parallel to the floor, engage your core and pull your hands toward your chest while keeping your elbows tight to your sides. Stop when your hands reach your chest and hold that position for 3–5 seconds. Slowly and carefully extend your arms straight out until your elbows are straightened but not locked, then push straight up through your heels back to a standing position.

That's 1 rep.

Wall Sit

While this motion is very similar to a squat, wall sits are a timed exercise. The goal is to increase your leg strength. This move is actually tougher than it seems and a good exercise to mix in with squats and lunges if you get bored.

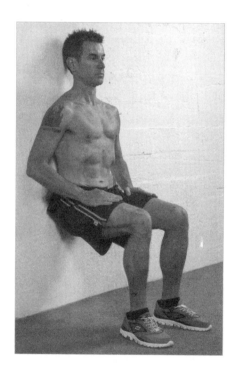

THE POSITION: Place your back flat against a stable wall and walk your feet out, sliding your back down the wall, until your upper and lower legs are at a 90° angle. Keeping your head up, core engaged and spine straight, breathe normally as you begin to count. You can place your hands on your thighs if you need extra support, let them hang by your sides, or raise them overhead or straight out.

BALL VARIATION: Place a stability ball between your back and the wall and perform a traditional wall sit. This really works a ton of connecting muscles in your lower body and core.

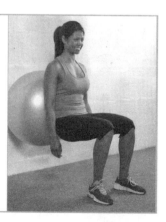

Squat

Squat form is crucial to getting the most out of this extremely beneficial exercise. Check out your form by using a full-body mirror and standing perpendicular to it as you complete your reps.

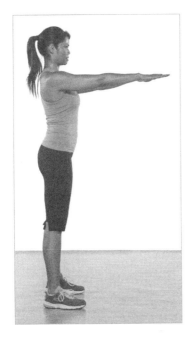

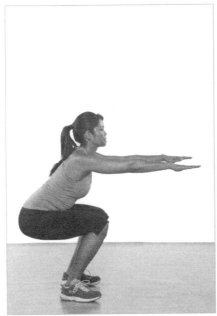

2 Bend at the hips and knees and "sit back" just a little bit as if you were about to sit directly down into a chair. Keep your head up, eyes forward and arms out in front of you for balance. As you descend, contract your glutes while your body leans forward slightly so that your shoulders are almost in line with your knees. Your knees should not extend past your toes and your weight should remain between the heel and the middle of your feet—do not roll up on the balls of your feet. Stop when your knees are at 90° and your thighs are parallel to the floor. If you feel your weight is on your toes or heels, adjust your posture and balance until your weight is in the middle of your feet.

Push straight up from your heels back to starting position. Don't lock your knees at the top of the exercise. This is 1 rep.

1 Stand tall with your feet shoulder-width apart and toes pointed slightly outward, about 11 and 1 o'clock. Raise your arms until they're parallel to the floor.

Forward Lunge

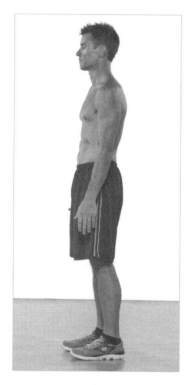

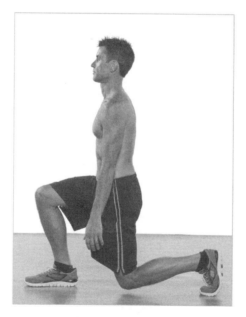

2 Take a large step forward with your right foot, bend both knees and drop your hips straight down until both knees are bent 90°. Your left knee should almost be touching the ground and your left toes are on the ground behind you. Keep your core engaged and your back, neck and hips straight at all times during this movement.

Pushing up with your right leg, straighten both knees and return to starting position. Repeat with the other leg.

1 Stand tall with your feet shoulder-width apart and your arms hanging at your sides.

REVERSE VARIATION: Reverse lunges are just like their forward counterparts, but begin by taking a step backward. These can be slightly more difficult to maintain your balance and are a bit better for activating supporting muscles in your pelvis, legs and core.

Warm-Ups

Arm Circle

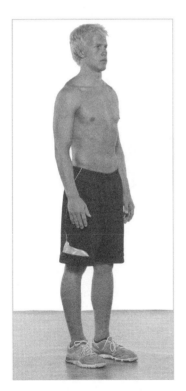 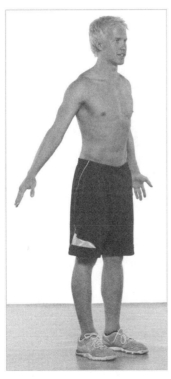 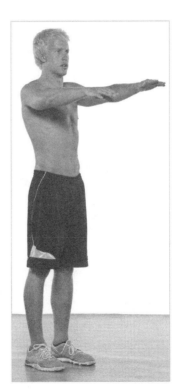

1 Stand with your feet shoulder-width apart.

2–3 Move both arms in a complete circle forward 5 times and then backward 5 times.

Neck Circle

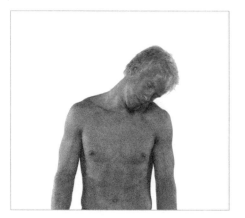

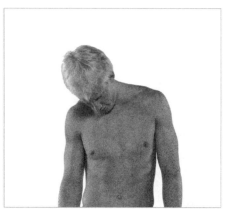

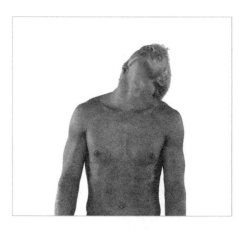

1 Standing like a soldier (with your back straight, shoulders square and chest raised), slowly lower your left ear to your left shoulder. To increase the stretch, you may use your left hand to gently pull your head toward your shoulder. Hold for 5–10 seconds.

2–3 Slowly roll your chin to your chest and then lower your right ear to right shoulder. Again, you may use your hand to enhance the stretch. Hold for 5–10 seconds.

Return your head to normal position and then tilt back slightly and look straight up. Hold for 5–10 seconds.

Lumber Jack

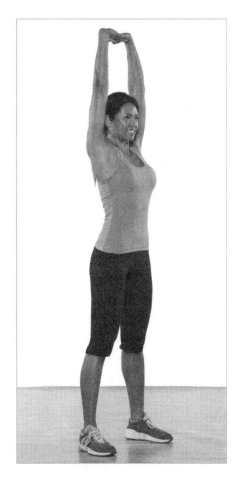

1 Stand with your feet shoulder-width apart and extend your hands overhead with elbows locked, fingers interlocked, and palms up.

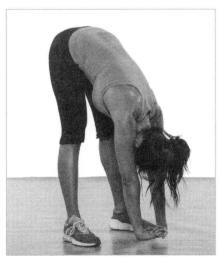

2 Bend forward at the waist and try to put your hands on the ground (like you're chopping wood). Raise up and repeat.

Around the World

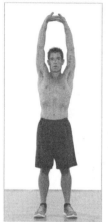
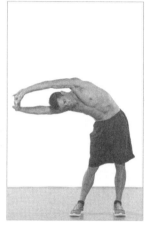
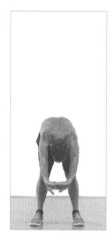

1 Stand with your feet shoulder-width apart and extend your hands overhead with elbows locked, fingers interlocked and palms up. Keep your arms straight the entire time.

2-3 Bending at the hips, bring your hands down toward your right leg, and in a continuous circular motion bring your hands toward your toes, then toward your left leg and then return your hands overhead and bend backward.

Repeat three times, then change directions.

Jumping Jacks

1 Stand tall with your feet together and arms extended along your sides, palms facing forward.

2 Jump 6–12 inches off the ground and simultaneously spread your feet apart an additional 20–30 inches while extending your hands directly overhead.

Jump 6–12 inches off the ground and return your hands and feet to starting position. Do 10 reps.

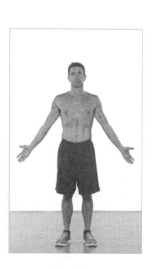
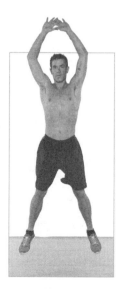

Jumping Rope

This exercise will work your legs, glutes and core and also tax your cardiovascular system to burn calories and fat.

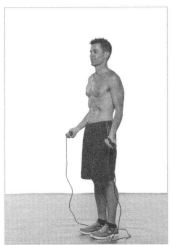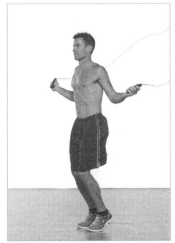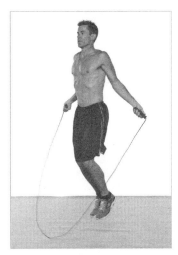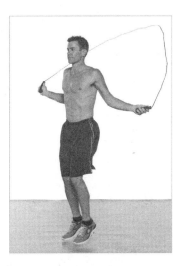

1 Stand erect with your feet shoulder-width apart, knees slightly bent and arms extended along your sides. Throughout the movement your weight should be distributed evenly on the balls of both feet. Grip the jump rope handles and extend the apex of the jump rope loop on the ground behind your feet.

2 Rotate your wrists forward to swing the rope overhead. The first movement from a dead stop will require more arm and shoulder movement, but as you progress on subsequent jumps, your arms should remain in a semi-static downward position along the sides of your body and your hands should rotate in small arcs.

3 As the apex of the rope's loop approaches the ground in front of your body and is 6 inches away from your toes, jump straight up approximately 4 to 6 inches off the floor with both feet as the rope passes underneath.

4 Land on the balls of both feet and bend your knees slightly to cushion the impact while continuing to rotate your wrists and swing the rope in an arc from back to front.

Stretches

Standing Hamstring Stretch

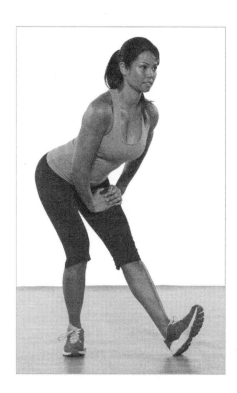

THE STRETCH: Stand with both feet together. Step your left foot forward 10 to 12 inches in front of your right foot with your heel on the floor and your toes lifted. With your abdominals engaged, bend your right knee slightly and lean forward from your hips, not your back or shoulders. You may need to rotate the toes of your right foot slightly outward to maintain balance and get a deep stretch. Keeping your shoulders back (don't round them to get a deeper stretch), place both hands on your left leg at the thigh and hold for 10–15 seconds.

Switch sides.

Standing Quad Stretch

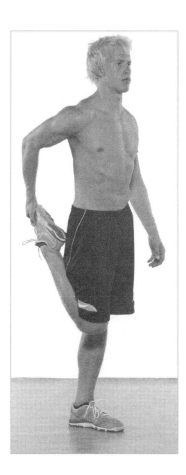

THE STRETCH: Stand with your feet hip-width apart. Bend your left leg and bring your left foot toward the bottom of your left buttock. Grasp your foot with your right hand, using your left hand to balance against a wall, desk or chair. With your knee pointed directly at the floor, gently pull your foot toward your butt until you find a position that stretches the front of your thigh. Hold that position for 10–15 seconds.

Switch sides.

Forearm & Wrist

Begin the stretch gently and allow your forearms to relax before stretching them to their full range of motion.

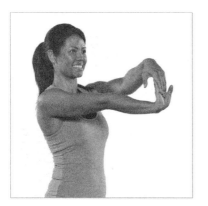 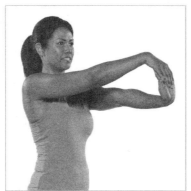

THE STRETCH: Stand with your feet shoulder-width apart and extend both arms straight out in front of you. Keep your back straight. Turn your right wrist to the sky and grasp your right fingers from below with your left hand. Slowly pull your fingers back toward your torso with your left hand; hold for 10 seconds.

Switch sides.

Shoulders

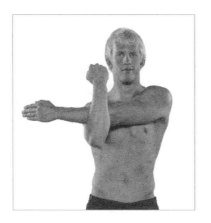 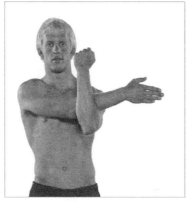

THE STRETCH: Stand with your feet shoulder-width apart and bring your left arm across your chest. Support your left elbow with the crook of your right arm by raising your right arm to 90°. Gently pull your left arm to your chest while maintaining proper posture (straight back, wide shoulders). Don't round or hunch your shoulders. Hold your arm to your chest for 10 seconds.

Release and switch arms. After you've done both sides, shake your hands out for 5–10 seconds.

Shoulders & Upper Back

1 Stand with your feet shoulder-width apart and extend both arms straight out in front of you. Interlace your fingers and turn your palms to face away from your body. Keep your back straight.

2 Reach your palms away from your body. Exhale as you push your palms straight out from your body by pushing through your shoulders and upper back. Allow your neck to bend naturally as you round your upper back. Continue to reach your hands and stretch for 10 seconds.

Rest for 30 seconds then repeat. After you've done the second set, shake your arms out for 10 seconds to your sides to return blood to the fingers and forearm muscles.

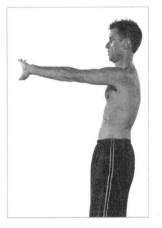 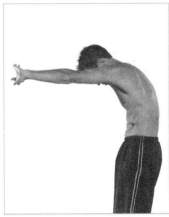

Chest

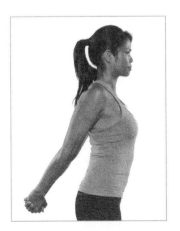

THE STRETCH: Clasp your hands together behind your lower back with palms facing each other. Keeping an erect posture and your arms as straight as possible, gently pull your arms away from your back, straight out behind you. Keep your shoulders down. Hold for 10 seconds.

Rest for 30 seconds and repeat.

Arms

THE STRETCH: Stand with your feet shoulder-width apart. Maintaining a straight back, grab your elbows with the opposite hand. Slowly raise your arms until they're slightly behind your head. Keeping your right hand on your left elbow, drop your left hand to the top of your right shoulder blade. Gently push your left elbow down with your right hand, and hold for 10 seconds.

Rest for 10 seconds and then repeat with opposite arms.

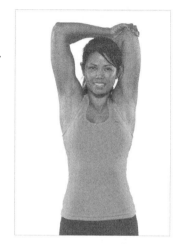

Child's Pose

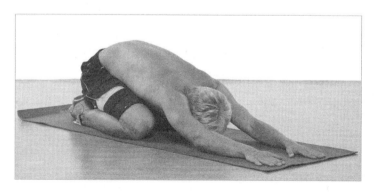

THE STRETCH: From a kneeling position, sit your butt back on your calves, then lean forward and place your lower torso on your thighs. Extend your arms directly out in front of you, parallel to each other, and lower your chest toward the floor. Reach your arms as far forward as you can, and rest your forearms and hands flat on the floor. Hold for 30 seconds. Release and then rest for 10 seconds.

Triathlon Terms

Following is a list of some common triathlon terms, and by no means is this an exhaustive list. Some of these terms are really important parts of the rules of triathlon (wetsuit-legal, drafting, blocking) and a handful are tongue-in-cheek references to things that happen out on the course. There are also quite a few bits of information that can be gleaned from the definitions; our goal is for you to learn something while you're chuckling along. For even more lingo you'll hear from triathletes, check out www.7weekstofitness.com.

Aero Bars   On triathlon-specific bikes, these extra handlebars are perpendicular to traditional "handlebars" (on triathlon bikes those are called "base bars") and they allow a rider to lean forward onto them to make their profile more aerodynamic. They hold the shifting levers for the front and rear derailleurs. Road bikes can quickly be retrofitted with a pair of clip-on aero bars.

Age-Grouper   Any non-professional triathlete. Age groups are usually broken into categories of every 5 years starting at 19 years of age.

Aid Station   During the run sections, aid stations are stocked with water and/or sports drinks. During triathlons longer than a sprint, energy gels and bananas are common. For long course and ultra distance events, the menu can include orange slices, chicken broth, flat cola and pretzels.

Athena and Clydesdale   Male athletes who weigh over 200 pounds qualify for the Clydesdale category, while the weight minimum for Athena classification in females is 145 pounds. Normally, there is an Open class for athletes 18 to 39 years old and a Master's class for athletes over 40.

Blocking   Riding to the left in such a manner that other cyclists cannot pass; this is an illegal move during the bike leg. Side-drafting, a form of blocking, is also illegal. See "Hell on Wheels: The Bike Course" on page 29 for passing rules during the bike course.

Body Glide/No-Chafe   Every experienced triathlete or marathoner will tell you, "Where skin touches skin, you will chafe." There are several products on the market that lubricate and provide protection from chafing; use them liberally and often, especially on the inner thighs, groin, butt and armpits.

Bonking   Generally refers to running out of energy on the bike or run, and in extreme cases can mean total-body shutdown.

Bottle drop   During the bike portion of most longer races, the aid stations are called bottle drops. Here you can swap out your empty water bottle for a new one or get a refill.

Brick   A training technique where you pick two disciplines from triathlon and perform them one after the other. For an example, a swim-run brick would consist of a swimming workout followed by a run. Both the training programs in this book feature brick workouts. The name "brick" is said to come from the way your legs feel after a particularly hard workout, and more commonly it's called a "building block" to your total triathlon fitness.

Cadence   On the bike, this is the number of times you turn the pedals (crank) per minute. Downhill or on a fast course, this can be over 120 rpm and uphill it can easily dip to half that amount.

Disc/Aero wheels   On the bike, these wind-cheating wheels reduce drag and help a cyclist ride faster. Anecdotal evidence points to 20 mph being the

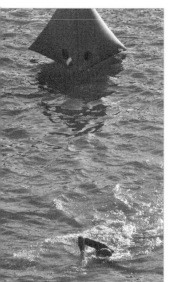

point at which rear solid disc wheels or deep-dished aero wheels begin to provide a distinct, legal advantage.

Doritos/Beach balls   The inflatable buoys that mark the turns during the swim portion.

Drafting   Following less than the distance of 7 meters (about 3 bike lengths) behind or within 2 meters next to another cyclist. This is illegal in all triathlons (except those deemed "draft-legal"). The rider who is drafting gets as much as a 40 percent reduction in wind resistance by positioning themselves in a low-pressure area directly behind the lead cyclist. When caught by an official, this will result in a time penalty. When caught by other riders, this will usually result in some choice words. Drafting is legal during the swim and on the run.

Getting aero   Positioning your body to be as streamlined as possible. Extending your arms on aero bars—dual bars extending from the center of the handlebars—allows you to get as low as possible, thereby reducing drag. While on the bike, it's important to become as aerodynamically efficient as possible to reduce wind drag and maintain speed.

Getting chicked   When a male triathlete is passed by a female triathlete. Used as a tongue-in-cheek phrase, strong female triathletes have been known to remember exactly how many men they "chicked" during a race.

Every male triathlete, from professionals to age-groupers, has been chicked at least once.

Getting on someone's feet   Drafting during the swim. This is completely legal, and the advantage of swimming in another swimmer's slipstream can yield as much as a 10 percent reduction in effort. The combined effect of the front swimmer's current and their kick oxygenating the water allows the drafting swimmer to swim faster with less exertion. Also, if you're confident this swimmer is appropriately swimming the course, your need to sight is reduced.

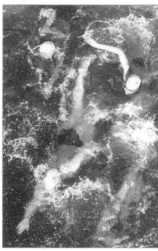

Legs   Swim, bike and run are the three sections, or "legs," of a triathlon, and normally performed in that order. Some races will swap the order around and will usually label the event a "reverse triathlon."

Loops   Many race courses have multiple loops on the bike and run, and less frequently it occurs on the swim. Normally, athletes will have to keep track of how many loops they have completed themselves, although some courses offer timing mats that count the number of revolutions for each racer.

M-Dot   A symbol taken from the Ironman logo, a dot on top of the letter M, which resembles a person.

According to WTC, It represents the need to have a fit body and a strong willpower. The M-Dot logo is trademarked by WTC, but is commonly seen as a tattoo on an Ironman finisher's calf.

Modesty tent   Gender-specific changing tents are provided for athletes to duck into and swap their clothes during transition. Some courses have 'em, some don't, but they're most common in long course and ultra-distance triathlons. Most professionals and fast age-groupers will skip the modesty tent and wear the same tri-suit for the entire race.

Mount/dismount line   Where racers can legally mount their bike after exiting via Bike Out. It's against the rules to mount or ride bikes in transition and will result in disqualification. When the bike leg is complete, the Dismount Line is where athletes get off and run their bikes until re-racking them at their spot in transition.

Newbies   First-timers, beginners or inexperienced triathletes.

Sighting   The act of viewing where you're going during the swim. It's harder than it looks. In pool swims, the lane lines and markers help keep you in a straight line; in open water, there are only buoys to show where to turn. These "Doritos" can be difficult to sight with other swimmers splashing around you. Newcomers will usually go slow and employ a breast stroke while raising their head out of the water, while the seasoned triathlete will

practice during training and make an efficient glimpse on the horizon as they take a breath.

Snot rockets   An affectionate term for the practice of covering one nostril and forcibly exhaling through the opposite nostril. While it's not the most attractive move, there's a certain art form to clearing one's nose while cycling or running without getting the projectile on your clothes or bike and it's more effective than wiping your nose on your shirt or bike glove. Snot rockets are performed to the right on the bike so as not to hit passing cyclists. On the run, make sure no one is in close proximity.

Strippers   The volunteers that help you remove your wetsuit after the swim. The process is pretty simple: Unzip your wetsuit as you run up to them and then sit on your butt for a second; they give it a tug from your shoulders and "ppfhwap!" it's off.

Swim In, Bike Out, Bike In and Run Out   The entrances and exits to the transition area and are usually clearly marked with signs or a large inflated archway. (See "Setting Up Your Transition Gear" on page 36.)

T1   Transition 1: After the swim, you enter the transition area and swap your wetsuit and goggles for cycling gear and run your bike to the mount line beyond the Bike Out transition exit.

T2   Transition 2: Post-cycling, get off the bike at the dismount line and run your bike through the Bike In entrance to the transition area. Re-rack your bike and change into your running gear, then exit via the Run Out.

Timing chip   Most triathlons feature a timing chip worn around the ankle that keeps track of each individual athlete's time based on their racer number. A timing chip is a passive radio frequency transponder that's "read" by antennas within timing mats placed on the ground. These timing mats are usually located in the entrances and exits of transition areas, as well as the finish line, and track each individual athlete's swim, transition 1, bike, transition 2 and run times. These times are referred to as "splits."

Transition   Where you rack your bike and store the gear you'll use for the bike and run; you'll normally have the swim gear on prior to the start of the race. (See "Setting Up Your Transition Gear" on page 36).

Tri bike   A triathlon-specific bike differs from a road bike in a myriad of ways. The seat tube, rake of the head tube, top tube and chainstays are all usually distinctly different lengths. The shape of tri bike downtubes are normally flatter and more aerodynamic, while road bike tubes are traditionally round. The more upright angle of a triathlon seat in relation to the handlebars is said to employ a pedaling style more similar to a runner, thereby providing an advantage to a true triathlete.

Tri shorts   Triathlon-specific shorts differ from traditional bike shorts in the size, shape, fit and consistency of the groin pad. While bike shorts usually feature a foam pad, triathlon shorts use a chamois. The former is famous for filling with water during the swim and looking and feeling like a full diaper afterward, while tri shorts are made to go from swim to bike to run.

Tri suit   Worn for all three legs of the race by experienced and pro triathletes, these extremely tight one- or two-piece suits are made out of space-age materials that have a low drag coefficient on the bike and run. Tri suits are made to be worn under a wetsuit; however, hydrodynamic "speed suits" are specific tri suits worn by experienced triathletes for races where wetsuits are not allowed.

Warming your wetsuit   Peeing in your wetsuit. Go ahead and giggle, nearly every triathlete will admit to doing it.

Washing machine   This is how the experience at the start and during the turns of a swim portion are usually described; hundreds of athletes trying to stroke and kick in a tight area. The splashing and limbs flying can result in some bumps and bruises, and is usually the cause of fear for many first-timers.

Wetsuit-legal   Prior to the start of each event, the water temperature will be checked to measure if it's below 78°F; if so, wetsuits are allowed for the swim portion of the race. For the most part, you're never required to wear a wetsuit unless it's an extreme event in very cold water. Wetsuits are never allowed in pool-based swims.

TRIATHLON RACE-DAY CHECKLIST

You can also download a printable version of this list at www.7weekstofitness.com.

PRE-/POST-RACE GEAR

- ❏ Warm Clothes/Jacket
- ❏ Sandals
- ❏ Cap/Visor
- ❏ Change of Clothes
- ❏ Pre-/Post-Race Nutrition

SWIM

- ❏ Swimsuit/Wetsuit
- ❏ Goggles

BIKE

- ❏ Bike (tuned, tires inflated)
- ❏ Bike Shoes
- ❏ Helmet
- ❏ Water Bottles
- ❏ On-Bike Nutrition (energy gels, bars)
- ❏ Sunglasses

RUN

- ❏ Shoes
- ❏ Socks (if necessary)
- ❏ Race Belt with Number
- ❏ Run Nutrition (energy gels, bars)

TRANSITION

- ❏ Sunscreen
- ❏ Anti-Chafe/Skin Lubricant
- ❏ Water Bottle
- ❏ Towel
- ❏ Shorts (if necessary)
- ❏ Shirt (if necessary)

Index

Acknowledgments

Thanks to Tri-Scottsdale, ONE Multisport, the ESPN Triathlon Team and HITS Triathlon Series. Without their help and support, this book would not have been possible. Special thanks to Tri for the Cure benefitting Susan G. Komen for the Cure, and to Preston Miller and Christina Catalano for their tireless help in pursuing a cure. A portion of the purchase price of this book goes to support Tri for the Cure. Learn more at www.triforthecureaz.com. —B.S. and L.E.

To Michael DeAngelo, Christopher Goggin, Erik and Mandy Mattheis, Jason Warner, Christopher Wilson, Scot Little, Matt Perkins and all of my multisport friends, thank you for making competing such a big part of my life. Special thanks to Mark H. Wilson of HITS Triathlon Series, Frank P. Sole of Sole Swim Solutions and Nick Clark of Clark Endurance. To Kristen and Vivi—thank you for teaching me that every time I come home I have truly won. —B.S.

To my father, Bill Elliot, for always presenting me with endless options and allowing me to make mistakes, which in turn allows me to truly own my successes. To my brothers, Porter and Blair, for being awesome, and putting up with my ridiculous competitive nature for the last 30 or so years. The Arizona Triathlon Community and all of my sponsors are beyond compare; without you guys I couldn't wake up and exercise all day, nor would I want to! Last, to my late mother, "Stevie," for all of her love and support that only a mother can give. —L.E.

About the Authors

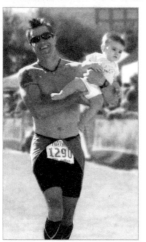

Brett Stewart is a National Council for Certified Personal Trainers (NCCPT)–certified personal trainer, a running and triathlon coach, and an endurance athlete who currently resides in Phoenix, Arizona. An avid multisport athlete and Ironman finisher, Brett has raced dozens of triathlons, multiple marathons and even a few ultra-marathons. To learn more about Brett's other books or to contact him, visit www.7weekstofitness.com.

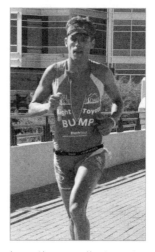

Lewis Elliot is a professional triathlete, coach, model and actor living in Scottsdale, Arizona. He has raced triathlon professionally since 2002, and prior to that was a US National Team Cyclist having won three US National Championships. Lewis has represented the USA in five World Championships, and has been the overall winner in over 150 multisport events. He has an Ironman personal best of 8 hours and 38 minutes.